E. Jean Alexander

Bloody Monday
Fibroid Tumors....My Ordeal

This book is based on a true story and all names in the book are fictitious. I began to capture my thoughts, feelings and frustration in a spiral note pad, during my endless waits in doctors' offices, the days taken off from work because of heavy bleeding and what seemed to be endless tiredness. After a few months the notepad I used was nearly full. One day when I was feeling okay, I transferred my feeling and thoughts from the notepad to the computer and was surprised that I had written over eighty pages. I decided with the encouragement of friends and family to complete and publish this book to tell my story, because so many women suffer from fibroid tumors.

For Information Contact:
AleCarn Publishing
P.O. Box 14454
Atlanta, Georgia 30324
Email: jalexander@alecarn.com
Website: www.alecarn.com

Library of Congress Control Number: 2001117815

ISBN 0-9711387-0-2

First Printing 2001

Printed in the U.S.A. by
Morris Publishing
3212 East Highway 30
Kearney, NE 68847
1-800-650-7888

My love and gratitude goes to my family for their love, endurance, and continued support. Without them it would have been harder to make the decisions about the course of treatment I chose.

To my dear friends, for months they listened to my one and only conversation, "Fibroids." I would also like to thank them for encouraging me to continue to write and publish this book. Thank you, from the deepest part of my heart.

Special Note To Readers

This book does not endorse any medical treatments, whether natural or traditional. Please consult with your physician to determine a course of treatment that is right for you. I strongly encourage all women and their families to take an active part in their choice of medical treatment for fibroid tumors.

Bloody Monday
Fibroid Tumors….My Ordeal

E. Jean Alexander

www.alecarn.com

It was late in the fall when I made an appointment with my primary doctor for a physical because I was feeling a little sluggish. I had blamed my tiredness on my new promotion. The position was somewhat stressful, and could be very demanding. I was hoping that the doctor would suggest a good vitamin to take.

I have been in good health most of my life, but I have to admit in the last few years, I have neglected to take good care of myself. I do try to get a physical at least once a year and my HMO primary doctor always encouraged me to get a Pap Smear and I just put it off.

I've had the usual female problems, cramps, and heavy bleeding in the last few years. I had also experienced PMS and a few other minor female problems.

As I sat in the examination room reading, the nurse came in asking questions.

"How are you Jean?"

"Oh, I'm okay. Well, I am not okay. I'm tired most of the time."

"Get on the table and let's take your temperature and blood pressure," she said.

"Is my blood pressure okay?" I inquired after she took the blood pressure cuff off my arm.

"Yes, it's fine, your temperature is okay too. You're here for a physical, so I will need you to take off everything and put on this gown with the opening in the back. The doctor will be in to see you shortly."

"Okay," I said as she walked out of the room.

I hate this part of the doctor's visit, pulling off my clothes. Wouldn't it be nice if we could be examined like they do on those science fiction TV programs? You don't have to take your clothes off. The doctor can tell exactly what's wrong with you by using this neat little medical scanner and fix the problem with a zap.

I took off my clothes and got back on the table. I wondered if I smelled clean. Somehow I never feel clean enough at the doctor's office. Having your clothes off with a paper gown opened in the back can be a little drafty. I tried to pull the one fit all gown around my back, but it didn't work. Why don't they make these gowns bigger for women like me?

Finally, I gave up struggling to cover my backside with the gown and turned my attention back to my book. I hope this will not be a long wait because my backside was quite drafty. It seemed sort of backward to wait in the waiting room and then you have another wait for the doctor in the examination room.

Just as I was settling back into the second chapter of my programming book, Dr. Konox walked in with my chart. He had such a soft and caring attitude as he flipped through my chart saying nothing.

"Well, I see you are in for a physical today. Is anything bothering you?" He asked.

"Well, I am tired most of the time." I said.

"Okay, lie back on the table and let's see what's going on." He said.

I am not much of a talker, I just did as the doctor ordered and in a few minutes the examination was complete.

"You said you were feeling tired. The last time you were here your periods were heavy. Are you still having heavy periods?"

"Yes, I am," I said.

I hate talking about these things, especially with men. I hoped by being short and to the point he would sense my feeling and change the subject.

"Well, I'll need to get a blood, and urine test, to see what's going on." He said as he wrote in my chart.

"Everything else looks okay. You do have an enlarged uterus. Have you had a Pap Smear this year?" He asked.

"No, but I plan to have one soon."

"Let me know when you have it done," he said.

"Okay, I will," I said.

"Take this to the nurse. She'll give you papers for lab tests. Come back here when you are complete." He instructed me.

I took my chart to the nurse and dreaded another wait in the lab. She gave me the paper and said, "Go to the second floor for your lab tests, and don't forget to come back here after the labs tests are completed."

I caught the elevator down to the second floor and to my surprise there wasn't anyone in the lab waiting room. As I put my paper in the tray and sat down, I was praying that the lab technician would get to me quickly and I could go back upstairs and find out what the tests results are, check out and get home early for once in a long time.

"Ms. Alexander, come on back, go to the bathroom and give me a urine sample. Use the cups and write your name on the cup and bring it to me when you are finished. When you come back have a seat in this chair," the lab technician said without catching her breath.

"Okay," I said.

Each time I give these urine samples, I always ponder whether to write my name on the cup before or after I deposit my sample. Again, I wondered why they didn't have waterproof labels to write your name on and then put the label on the cup. What if I wasted the urine sample trying to write my name on the cup? I wrote my name on the cup without incident, using the permanent marker and went back to the Lab to have a blood sample taken.

"Which arm do you want me to take the blood from?" the lab technician asked.

"It doesn't matter," I said.

Either way it is going to hurt. I thought as I rolled up my sleeves. I hope she is good at this. I hope it doesn't hurt. I looked up at the ceiling as she drew the blood from my arm.

"Okay, I'll need to get one more tube and we'll be finished." She said.

Good we are finished. It looks like I am going to get out of this place in record time after all. One hour and counting. One hour and counting. I took the elevator back to the doctor's office and gave the lab sheet to the nurse.

"Will I have to wait long?" I asked her.

"No, let me take this back to the doctor and he will come out and let you know about the urine test. The blood test will come back in a few days, and we'll call you with those results," she said.

She took the lab papers back to the doctor and I went back to the waiting room to wait again. It would be nice if you could get your blood test, urine test and all of those things done when you first arrived. That would save a little time.

While waiting, I tried leafing through some of the magazines, but none of them interested me. I tried studying my programming book, but that did not help either. I was eager to hear what the doctor had to say and then I just wanted to go home. I would not find out about why I am feeling tired until the blood tests came back in a few days anyway.

I was fretting after fifteen minutes passed and still the doctor had not come to tell me about the test. Finally after about twenty minutes, he put his head in the door. He looked around and found that I was the only one in the waiting room. The doctor sat down beside me and told me that I had a urinary tract infection. He gave me a prescription for the urinary tract infection and told me he would have the nurse call about the blood test.

"Take care of yourself," he said.

"I will," I replied.

At this point, I was not so concerned with how I felt, I just wanted to get out of the doctor's office and go home. I checked out at the front desk and the medical clerk informed me about my next appointment.

"The doctor wants to see you in two weeks. We do have something available. Do you want to make the appointment now, about the same time?"

"Yes, that will be okay. I like coming in the late afternoon," I said.

"Okay, we'll see you in two weeks." She said and gave me an appointment card. I gave her my co-pay and got my receipt. Oh, at last it was good to get out of here.

A few days later Dr. Konox's nurse called and told me that I was anemic. My red blood count was very low and that was causing me to feel tired all the time.

"The doctor have prescribed some iron pills for you to take. Take them according to the instruction on the label." She said.

She asked me about calling in the prescription to the drug store. I gave her the drug store's number, and told her to have a good day.

This was simple enough. I will take the iron pills and the pills to cure the urinary tract infection and then I will begin to feel better. The next day I picked up the iron pills from the pharmacy, and began to take them that day alone with my regular vitamins. In a few days I did begin to feel better. I was still feeling tired, but not to the point where I was just glad to see the bed when I got home everyday.

I went back to the doctor in two weeks to have my finger pricked for a blood count. My blood count was up. I was pleased with the results the iron pills had made.

Bloody Monday Fibroid Tumors....My Ordeal

A week later my period came on. It was very heavy and I felt exhausted after the second day. I continued to take the iron pills. After a few days, I was feeling better, but a little weak and tired. I was concerned with why I bled so heavily each month.

I went back to the doctor and found that my blood count had gone down again. The doctor showed concern and again asked me had I visited my gynecologist. I told him no. He advised me that I needed to see my gynecologist for a Pap smear, or he could do the Pap Smear if it was okay with me.

I assured him that I would see the gynecologist. I didn't want him giving me a Pap Smear. He was my primary doctor. The doctor told me to continue taking the iron pills to get my blood count back up. I was taking fifteen grams of iron a day, and it was upsetting my stomach.

During the next few months, I was taking at least one day a month off from work because of heavy menstrual bleeding. I talked to a friend about my problem, and to my surprise she had the same problem. She told me about the herbs she was taking to help relieve the symptoms.

"You know my doctor is giving me fifteen grams of iron a day. He says my blood count is so low that he didn't know how I was functioning. All of that iron is upsetting stomach." I told her.

"Look I have to do the same thing, but I am doing something else also. I have been taking herbs to help me during that time of the month. Taking Kelp and Parsley helps a lot. I also take all of the "B" vitamins along with vitamin E." She said.

"I am going to try it. As soon as we leave here I am going to the Herb store and I am going to buy the Kelp and the Parsley." I said excitingly. I felt a glimmer of hope. Maybe this will help.

After I left her, I went to the herb store, and got the vitamins. I could not find the parsley, but I did find everything else. I began taking the vitamins and herbs immediately.

I waited patiently for my next month cycle. It was not as heavy as it usually is and I did not have to miss a day out of work. I called my friend and told her that I had a good month.

I thanked my friend over and over for the advice and decided to stick with it. Several months went by and the most I experienced was the second day that was a little heavy, but nothing to stay at home for. Oh, I wish I had been doing this all along. I did not know that a few herbs and some vitamins could have such great results.

I called my doctor and told him that the iron he prescribed was too harsh for my stomach. After I finished taking the iron he prescribed, I decided to take a smaller amount of iron in an over the counter form.

Bloody Monday Fibroid Tumors....My Ordeal

Almost a year went by and everything appeared to be okay. There was only one thing. I always wondered why I could not pull my stomach all the way in. I use to be able to do this. I reasoned with myself. You are over forty Jean! I dismissed the thought of having a bigger stomach and contributed it to the so-called middle age spread.

One day I was looking at one of the Public Broadcasting stations. They were running one of their campaigns and I was very interested in the speaker. He was talking about taking a healthy approach to making changes in your lifestyle.

I called the station with my pledge because I wanted the book. The station was offering the health book as a gift for pledges of $75.00 or more. This sounded good. The speaker talked about being tired and what to eat and take to make you feel better. Most of the things he talked about using were natural foods, vitamins, and herbs. I was beginning to take more interest in taking a healthy and natural approach to my eating habits.

The next week I went to lunch with a friend from work and we went to the bookstore. To my surprise the book was there. I purchased it. I also made a donation to the Public Television station, because this is where I heard about this wonderful book.

I took the book home and began to read it. It was a very large book and as I flipped from page to page, I was wondering if I would ever get through it. I am not much of a reader, but this book caught by attention and I went to sleep reading it. The next day I had read almost half of the book. I was encouraged to start taking better care of myself.

I had not gone to the gynecologist as I had promised my primary doctor. The very next day I decided to make an appointment with the doctor. I called the gynecologist my daughter was seeing. She was booked until the middle of the following month. The nurse sent me a first visit package to fill out, so all of this would be complete when I came for my office visit. I thought about calling my regular gynecologist, but he had moved and the drive to see him was just too far.

I needed to see someone sooner, I reasoned. One of my co-workers and I were talking about female ailments and I asked her about her doctor. She told me and gave me her doctor's phone number.

"Oh good. She's not that far from work. Thank you." I told her.

I called for an appointment, and was told the doctor could see me on June 9th, at 9:30 a.m. This was just a week from today. I think I will go see her. I really did not want to wait a month to see the other doctor. I was pleased to know that I would be able to see the new doctor so soon.

I was really feeling good about myself. The vitamins appeared to be doing wonders, and every month I felt really good. The bleeding was still heavy on the second day, but after that it was manageable.

Little did I know the worst was yet to come. I could hardly wait until that Friday to see the doctor. I really wanted to know what my blood count was and if I had any other unknown problems. Friday morning finally came. The doctor's office was located in a hospital medical complex. Not being very good with directions, I missed my street and had to turn around which would surely make me late.

Bloody Monday Fibroid Tumors....My Ordeal

"Oh no, I'm going to be late." I said out loud as I looked at my watch and realized that I had only a few minutes to get to the office.

I hope no one was looking at me talking to myself. I really need to learn my way around this city. I have been here over twenty years and still get lost on the Peachtree Streets.

As I pulled into the parking lot, I became a little nervous. I had not been to the gynecologist in such a long time. I looked around and started to think. All of these people are sick!

Well, I am just going for a checkup! I made my way to the elevator and up to the seventh floor and to the doctor's office. I walked to the front desk and signed in.

"Have you been here before?" The receptionist asked.

"No, I have not." I replied.

"What doctor are you here to see?" She asked.

"I am here to see Dr. Barks. I replied.

"Okay, fill out this paperwork and bring it back to me." She instructed.

I found a seat, and before filling out the paperwork, I looked around and so many pregnant women.

Was I that big when I was pregnant? How did I survive being only five feet one half inch tall with such a big stomach?

I looked down at the paper I had to fill out and looked back up as one of the expectant mothers in slip on shoes pushed off the chair and headed for the bathroom.

Well, let me get through this paperwork, I thought. These women will have these babies soon and they will not be pregnant in a few months. I had several pages to fill out.
I finished the paperwork and gave it to the nurse along with my insurance card.

The nurse copied the insurance card and gave it back to me. I returned to my seat and wondered how long it would take to be seen by the doctor.

Well, I might as well get comfortable. I pulled out my book and began to read. I went through the first chapter and started on the second chapter when the nurse called my name.

"Ms. Alexander." She said in a loud voice.

I got up and followed the nurse back to another waiting room near the lab.

"Let's get your weight. Step on the scale." She said.

"Okay. Let me pull off my shoes. I don't want to weigh more than I have to." I said.

After I weighed in, I was asked to give a urine specimen and then I was shown to another waiting room. How many waiting rooms does this place have? I thought I was going to see the doctor. There were about four other women waiting to see the doctor. I had already been here an hour and still had not seen the doctor. Finally after another twenty minutes, another nurse called me to follow her.

"Let's get some blood from your finger to check your blood count." She said.

This is what I had been waiting for. I wanted to know what my blood count was. I wanted to see if all of the vitamins and herbs I was taking were working. I closed my eyes as the nurse pricked my finger and squeezed the blood from it. She put the small tube in a machine and turned it on.

"Okay, now let's get your blood pressure." She said.

After she finished taking my blood pressure, the nurse took me to a room and I was instructed to pull off my clothes.

"The doctor will be with you soon." She said as she walked out of the door.

Here we go with this clothes routine again. I began to pull my clothes off and put on the gown. I got on the table and began to read my book again. I wonder how long I am going to have to sit on this cold hard paper with the drafty paper gown opened in the back, until the doctor comes in.

It would really be nice if they could have some music playing or maybe a TV on the wall in these examination and waiting rooms. It would make the time go by faster. I sat on the end of the exam table and was swinging my legs when the doctor came in.

"Hello, Ms. Alexander, my name is Dr. Barks." She said with an accent.

"Hi." I said.

I was trying to figure out what country she may be from when she continued to speak.

"What type of problem are you experiencing?" She asked.

"I am here for a Pap Smear, breast exam and just a normal checkup. I do have a slight itching problem from time to time." I told her.

"Is this itching before or after your period?" She asked.

"Well, I get it after my period. I use the over the counter cream, but I am still having some discomfort." I told her.

"Well, it could be yeast, or it could be a bacterial infection. If it is bacterial it may be appearing because of your cycle. There's not much we can do about that except to treat it on a monthly basis." She explained.

" Okay." I answered.

"Okay, let's examine you and get a Pap Smear. I will also get a specimen and check for yeast and bacterial okay? Just relax and we will be finished in a minute." She said.

"When was the last time you had a Pap smear and mammogram?" She asked.

"Oh, it's been a few years." I replied.

"Well, we will have to correct that. It looks like you are here for a checkup just to see if everything is working okay." She laughed.

"Yes, I am. I have neglected that for the last two years. However, I do see my primary doctor yearly." I told her.

She's very pleasant. I thought to myself as I tried to take my mind off the examination. I don't like being examined, but this doctor was gentle and she was very good at her job.

"Ms. Alexander, you have two very large fibroids. They appear to be about as big as an orange. One is a little smaller than the other. Did you know you have them?" She asked.

"Yes, I do." I said.

"Are you having any problems with them?" She asked with concern in her voice.

"No I am not. " I said.

"Okay, we're finished. Let me take this to the lab. You can put your clothes back on, and I will be back in a minute" She said.

I would also like you to have an ultrasound to see exactly how large the fibroids are. I would also like you to have a mammogram. The nurse will give you the information on how to schedule these." She continued.

"Okay." I said.

The doctor left the room with the specimens. I got dressed and waited for her to return with the test results. After about fifteen minutes she returned.

"Well, your blood count is 44, and that is really good. Your blood pressure is also good." She said.

“Oh, that’s good.” I said.

I was really happy that the vitamins I was talking had worked. I was elated! Finally, I had done something right for my body.

“You do have a bladder infection. I did not find a bacterial infection but I did find a slight yeast infection. I have two prescriptions for you to take care of these problems. Other than that everything seems to be fine.” She looked at me and smiled.

“Oh, that’s great.” I said.

“I would like to see you in six weeks after you have completed the ultrasound and the mammogram. Take this information to the check out desk. Take care of yourself.” She said.

“Thanks.” I said.

I was happy I had only minor problems. I felt good, the fibroids were large, but they were not giving me any problems, so I thought. I was thankful and made myself a promise that I would not neglect my health again.

Finally, it’s over! I went to the check out desk and made my appointment to see the doctor in six weeks, and paid my co-payment. I went to another desk to make an appointment for an ultrasound to see how large the fibroids were. I also got information on where to call to schedule to have the mammogram done. I left the doctor’s office feeling good about myself. When I got to my car, I called my daughter and told her that my blood count was excellent.

Bloody Monday Fibroid Tumors....My Ordeal

"You laughed at me for taking all of those vitamins and herbs, but it paid off!" I screamed into the phone.

"That's good." She said.

"I'm headed for work, so I'll see you at the home." I told her.

The following week I was going on vacation. I needed to get some things finished, before I went on vacation. I was headed to Tennessee, and Mississippi to see my family and to do business.

This would not only be a vacation, it would be a working vacation. I would spend about three days presenting a network and website design to a company that I was working for. In order to do the work it would require me to be present on site.

I was not too thrilled about doing the site visit, because the site was in a remote location. But, I had made a commitment and I would follow through.

When I left work that Friday, I came home and continued to work on the design for the rest of the weekend for the presentation on the following Tuesday.

I felt a slight pain in my right side and it was becoming more uncomfortable as I sat at the computer to complete the designs.

By Saturday, the pain had backed off and I was looking at airline tickets. I called my contact in Tennessee and advised them that I would be arriving on Monday evening at about 5:30 p.m. I wanted to make sure that they would pick me up at the airport on time.

I spent most of the night online getting quotes for network servers, computers, and software for the project. I also completed the layout for the web page. This was one of the biggest projects I had ever been involved in. I wanted everything to be prefect or at least near perfect.

It was about 2:00 a.m. on Sunday morning when I finally had the quotes and the presentation for the project complete. I got up from the computer and felt this awful pain in my side.

"Ah, what is this?" I murmured to myself.

As I headed for the bathroom, the pain became more intense. I stopped and sat on the bed for a while. I held my side rubbing it, trying to detect if it was a bruise or something.

I prepared for bed. I had a pretty restful night, and by the next morning the pain was gone again. The rest of the day was filled with preparing for my flight on Monday. I was excited. If this deal goes through, I could maybe retire early? Everything was prepared and I was ready to spend a week presenting the project, Web site design and the estimated cost.

7:00 a.m. Monday morning I felt great. The pain was gone and I was telling my children my plans and when I would be back in town. Around 8:00 a.m. I felt a slight pain in my side.

"Oh, no not again!" I grasped as I grabbed my right side.

The pain at this point was sharp and I could not ignore it. It was getting worst by the minute. At this point I made a decision not to get on that plane to Tennessee. I felt crushed. I had worked so hard on this project, but I could not ignore the fact that I had this pain and I was feeling very sick. I did not call my brother, hoping that I could see the doctor and it would be nothing and I could still somehow make the evening flight. Deep inside I knew that I would not be making this trip at all.

I remembered that my primary doctor had sent me a letter informing me that he had moved from his downtown location to an area on the North side of town. It was off Georgia 400! This had to be the worst place to try and see the doctor early in the morning. I had the letter the doctor sent somewhere, but I couldn't find it. Finally, I remembered that I had put it in my briefcase. The pain was getting worst. I finally found the number. I called and listened as the recording finally told me what number to press to speak to my doctor's assistant.

"Dr Konox's office, this is Sue. How may I help you today?" She asked in a cheerful voice.

"Sue this is Jean Alexander, Do you have an appointment available for Dr. Konox today?" I asked.

"Let me see. No I don't. What's the problem?" She asked.

" I am having this awful pain in my right side. I've had it on and off since Friday, but today it is worst than any of the other days." I explained to her catching my breath, as the pain in my side got worst.

"Okay, let's see if we can work you in. Can you get in here by noon?" She asked.

"Yes, I can. Can you give me directions on how to get to the new office?" I asked her.

The receptionist gave me directions to the office explaining to me that this was a work in appointment and I may have to wait. Well, this is one thing that I am used to, waiting. At this point the pain was so sharp that it did not matter what the wait would be in the doctor's office. I was in serious pain. I called my daughter and told her that she would have to go to the doctor with me because I couldn't leave her at home alone.

Bloody Monday Fibroid Tumors....My Ordeal

I called my husband at work and told him I would be at the doctor's office. I told him about the pain that I was experiencing in my side.

As we were driving to the doctor's office the pain appeared to get better. When we pulled into the parking lot and got out of the car, I felt the pain return. It appeared to be worst than earlier in the day.

"Remember where we are parked. You know I am bad on remembering where I park the car." I joked with my daughter. I leaned over a little, and touched the side of my body where the pain was.

"I'll remember where we are parked Mama. Are you okay?" She asked.

I touched her head. "Yeah, I'm okay. I just need to see the doctor to see what's hurting inside me."

We found the doctor's office and I signed in at the front desk. As usual there were lots of forms to fill out and insurance to verify. I completed all of the forms and gave them to the receptionist. I was actually feeling better.

My daughter and I passed the time looking at a popular fashion magazine. I tried to be chipper, but the pain was coming back again. I hope it is not my appendix. My husband had this problem a few years ago and spent a week in the hospital, after it was taken out. The next year he had some additional complications and spent more than fourteen days in the hospital. I shuttered to think that I would have to go through the same thing.

My daughter continued to show me clothes in the fashion magazine. Although I could not concentrate on the magazine, I did make comments on what she showed me. I twisted and turned in the chair from the pain. I was trying hard not to show the pain that I was feeling in my facial expression. About 30 minutes later the nurse called my name.

"That was quick," I told her.

I looked at my daughter. " Be good and stay here until I get back."

"Okay," she replied, never looking up from the fashion magazine.

The nurse weighed me, got a urine specimen and took me to the exam room.

"Okay Jean, let's get your temp and blood pressure," She said.

"Okay," I replied.

"What seems to be the problem today?" She asked.

"I am having sharp pains in my right side," I told her.

As she wrote all of this information down in my chart, we chatted about the pain and what it could possibly be. She instructed me to undress down to my underwear and put on the famous open in the back paper gown. If the doctor is checking everything in the front, why do they want you to have the gown opened in the back? It would make more sense to have the gown open in the front. Of course it would have to be bigger for women like me.

After the nurse finished writing in my chart, she left the room. I did as she instructed, and picked up one of the magazine in the exam room and began to flip through the pages. I hope this will not be a long wait. I was thinking to myself. Just as I was reaching for another magazine, the doctor walked into the room.

"Hi Jean. What seems to be bothering you today?" He asked.

"I have this pain in my right side," I told him.

The doctor asked me a series of questions about the pain. He wanted to know if it moved when I changed positions. He wanted to know if the pain was in my back, or radiated to the left side of my body. I explained to him that none of these things were happening. The pain was only in my right side.

"It doesn't sound like your appendix is having problems," he said.

He went on to say, "Have you had your Pap Smear?"

"Yes, just last week. I had a complete exam by my gynecologist. I have not received the results from all of the tests, but the doctor said everything else looked okay." I told him.

The doctor continued to exam me. Then he said the most dreaded words.

"I am going to have to do a pelvic exam," he said.

I sat up on the table. “You do?” I asked him.

“Well, I need to know what’s going on. It doesn’t appear to be an appendix problem. I need to check to see if there is something else causing the problem,” he said in a kind, gentle voice.

The doctor began to give the nurse instructions on the instruments he would need for the pelvic examination. I was looking as she prepared the tools used for pelvic exams. I noticed that the pelvic examination tool had a light on it.

“Oh, they come with lights now.” I commented to the nurse.

“Yes they do. These are a lot better than the old ones. There is no need to have that big O’ bright light shining on you. This way the doctor can see inside you better while he’s examining you,” she grinned.

The nurse helped me get into position on the exam table. Oh, I hate these exams. My mind went back to the science fiction programs and the simple scanning tool used to examine you. I wonder will we ever get that technologically advanced. The doctor moved into position and the examination began!

“Everything looks okay.” The doctor said.

“Yeah, that’s what my gynecologist said,” I replied.

“Jean your uterus is very large. Did you know you have fibroids?” He asked.

“Yes, I do, but I haven’t had any problems with them. I’ve had them for over twenty years. I found out after the birth of my second child,” I told the doctor.

"Well, they are very large, about the size of oranges. One is a little smaller. You have two of them as far as I can tell." He continued to talk.

"Yes, I know." I responded to the doctor.

It was nice that he was talking while he was examining me. It put me more at ease. Still I would be glad when was he finished.

"Jean, these fibroids could be causing the pain in your side. Most of the other areas have been ruled out. Your urine test came back okay." He said in a serious tone.

The doctor continued to talk. "Just to be sure, I would like to get an ultrasound to totally rule our the appendix, and to see how large the fibroids are, and if they are causing your problem. I am also going to order a complete blood work up."

I was thinking, he has never talked this much. He has always been attentive to his patients, but today he seemed more concerned than normal. I could not help but think that something was seriously wrong.

The doctor began to speak again. "I'll make the arrangements for the ultrasound at the hospital. I'll call over now, because I think they will be closing soon." He said as he gave the nurse instructions to prepare me for the ultrasound tests.

"Okay Jean, you can get dressed now. To take the ultra sound you will have to drink at least 60 ounces of water to get your bladder full," she said.

"60 ounces of water now?" I asked her.

"Yep. I'm afraid so. Oh, I can't find the cups. I thought I had some cups here. Let me go and find you a paper cup," she said.

I thought about my daughter sitting in the waiting room. She must be tired by now.

The nurse came back into the exam room with the cup. She began to talk about some of the female problems she had experienced. They were very similar to the ones that I was beginning to experience. She told me about the operation she had to remove her uterus because of heavy bleeding, and how much better she felt.

"Okay, this is a six ounce cup. So, you will need to drink at least 10 of these. I'll be back in a few minutes." She instructed me as she left the room.

I began filling the cup and counting as I drank cup after cup of water. When I got to the ninth cup, I could feel my bladder filling up. The last cup of water somehow seemed warmer. I managed to get down the last six ounces of water. At this point, I was really feeling full. I leaned over the sink. My bladder felt like it was going to burst! I sat in the chair and waited for the nurse to come back in the room. My bladder was so full that I felt if I stood up, I would have this urge to go to the bathroom.

The nurse came back into the room. "Did you drink all ten cups of water?" She asked me.

"Yeah, I have." I told her.

"Okay let's go have the tests done," she said.

"Wait, I need to get my daughter. She's in the waiting room," I told her.

I went to the waiting room and waved for my daughter to come with me.

"Are we ready to go?" She asked.

"No, I have to have an ultrasound done. As soon as that is completed we will be going home. Thanks sweetie for being so patience." I told her as I touched her shoulder.

I felt like I had swallowed a basketball as I very slowly walked down the hall to the ultrasound lab in the hospital. I could feel the water in my bladder move as I walked into the waiting room.

I signed in and was waiting, when Dr. Konox showed up. He came over to where I was sitting.

"Jean, I need to get your blood work up before our lab closes." He said.

"Wait here a minute, let me go and see if they will wait a few minutes while you go to our lab for the blood tests" He instructed me as he went over to the receptionist desk.

The doctor asked if I could go back over to his office and have the blood tests done. He also asked the receptionist if they would wait until I got back to have the ultrasound test done.

"I am only doing this for you Dr. Konox. We'll wait until she finishes with the tests," the receptionist said.

"Okay Jean let's go get those tests done." The doctor said.

I instructed my daughter. "Wait here until I get back."

She looked up at me and said. "I wish I had brought my book."

The doctor and I left the ultrasound waiting room and he was walking fast.

I called out to him. "My bladder is full. I can't walk that fast. Wait for me."

"Oh, I'm sorry. We are here now," he said.

I sit down in the waiting room in the lab, as the doctor gave my paper work to the lab technician. This should only take a few minutes, and there is only one person ahead of me. I tried to sit as still as possible. There were twins in the waiting room and I was playing with them. This distracted me a little, and took my mind off the discomfort I felt.

The lab technician was complaining about having additional patients so close to closing time.

"It's time for me to go," he said as he looked up to see that he had two additional patients.

I just looked at him and did not make any remarks. If you felt the way I do you wouldn't be complaining about pricking someone's arm for blood I thought. I was becoming irritated. I had been waiting for more than 15 minutes. My side was hurting, and I had a bladder with 60 ounces of water about to burst. What is he doing to her arm? I thought to myself. It doesn't take that long to draw blood. She had been in there at least 10 minutes. When your bladder is full to capacity, a minute is a long time. I was looking at the ceiling, when the technician called my name.

"Ms. Alexander, come on back," he said.

I sit in the chair and watched as the lab technician typed on the keyboard.

"Your information is not in the computer. Do you have your insurance card?" He asked me.

Oh no, please hurry. If you don't hurry, you are going to have a very wet lab floor. I thought as I pulled out my card and gave it to him without saying a word. It appeared to me that he was taking his time typing the information. At last he finished typing and began to draw the blood from my arm.

"Okay Ms. Alexander, we're finished." He said.

"Thanks." I murmured.

Now I had to walk back to the ultrasound lab! My back was hurting, and I was walking even slower. I hope I can hold onto this water. The lab was not that far away, but it seemed like miles. Each step I took was an effort. The nurse saw me as I wobbled into the waiting room.

"Ms. Alexander, come on back. I know you are heavy with that water. I see you are walking kind of funny," she said in a cheerful voice.

"Yea." I managed a smile.

"Well, this won't take long." She assured me.

She showed me into the exam room and I undressed from the waist down to have the ultrasound done.

The technician picked up my chart and said. "We're here to see how large your fibroids are. Okay, this gel I am going to put on you will be a little cold," she warned me.

"Okay." I said.

I did not have much to say. My goal was to get though this as quickly as possible. So, I was going to cooperate completely. The nurse put the gel on my stomach and sides and began to run the probe over my stomach and sides.

"Do you see anything?" I asked her.

"Yes. You have some huge fibroids," she said.

The radiologist walked into the room and was talking to the technician about the size of the fibroids.

"Everything is looking okay, Ms. Alexander." The radiologist said and walked back out of the room.

It appeared that the technician was not as experienced at doing these tests as I thought she should have been. But, what do I know about doing ultrasounds? I have had an ultrasound before, and I know that they printed out the images. I had not heard the printer print anything.

"Do you see anything yet?" I asked the technician again.

"We have some good pictures. I will be printing them out.... Right now," she said.

"I am about to burst!"

"Okay," she said.

It took her a few more minutes to print out all of the images. Finally she said. "You can go to the bathroom now. Come back in here when you are finished."

She assisted me off the table and pointed me in the direction of the bathroom. I ran to the bathroom. I do not have to tell you how I felt. At this point going to the bathroom was more precious than gold. I went back into the exam room thinking that I could put my clothes back on, go home and wait for the doctor to give me the results of the ultrasound and blood tests in a few days. Wishful thinking!

"Jean, I don't know if you are aware of this, but we have two ways of doing ultrasounds. One is what we just finished with the bladder full. The other is vaginal with the bladder empty. This allows us to get a closer look at the ovaries and the rest of your female organs." She said.

"You mean we are not finished?" I asked her.

"Not yet, but we will be finished shortly." She instructed me.

I was looking as she prepared to do the second ultrasound. She pulled out this long round probe. That thing had to be at least 18 or more inches long!

"You're not going to put all of that inside me are you?" I asked her in a serious tone.

"I promise you, it will not hurt. If it does hurt just let me know okay." The technician assured me.

The second ultrasound test began. This one was more embarrassing and uncomfortable than the first ultrasound test.

"Oh Yes, these are some good images." The technician said as she moved the probe around in my body and printed out the images.

"Your bladder is filling up again, and I need you to empty it again," she said.

I got off the table and went to the bathroom and emptied my bladder again. I will be so glad when this is over. I thought as I walked back into the exam room and got back on the table. The technician put the long probe back in me and took a few more images and printed them out.

The Radiologist came back into the room, and looked at the images. "Ms. Alexander, I read your chart and saw that you are having some pain in your side. I just wanted to assure you that from your ultrasound tests there is not a life threatening condition present."

"Oh good," I said.

"Well, I didn't want you to be worried when you went home. However, you do have two huge fibroids. They are about the size of a four month fetus, or as large as an orange. This could be causing the pain. Other than that, the tests appear to be okay. You may want to look into treatment for these fibroids. We will take a further look at the images and consult with Dr. Konox on the final results," she said.

"Thank you." I said relieved.

"We're finished. You can get dressed." The technician told me.

"Thank you for everything." I told her.

"Oh, you are welcome. Your doctor will call you in a few days with the full results." She informed me. The Radiologist and the technician left the room and at last I felt as if the day had ended. Finally, I can go home! I got dressed in a hurry, and went out to the waiting room to get my daughter. She looked really tired.

"Let's go." I told her.

She did not say much as we walked to the parking lot. Today I remembered where I was parked! Maybe all that testing cleared my head. As we were leaving out of the parking lot I saw the technician crossing the street. She recognized me and waved. I waved back at her and smiled. It was so good to be going home. I looked at the clock and it was 7:00 p.m. I called my husband and told him that we were coming home.

"Do you need me to pick you up?" He asked.

"No. I 'm okay. You all go on to the meeting without us." I told him that our daughter and I would not be able to make it to the meeting.

"Okay, call me if you need anything. Are you sure you are okay?" He asked.

"Yes, I am okay." I assured him.

I really did not feel like cooking. It's amazing how women think. Even when we are sick we think about feeding and taking care of our families, before we take care of ourselves. I stopped by a fast food place and got dinner. I would not be cooking tonight.

Everything went okay that night. The pain was not as bad as it had been during the earlier part of the day. I had completely forgotten about my trip to Tennessee. I was exhausted. It had been a long day without a clear explanation of what was really causing the pain. The doctor did not prescribe anything for the pain except over the counter pain medicine.

"Oh dear, I need to call my brother." I cried out loud.

"Well, call him," my daughter said. I think she was more interested in eating the food we had picked up.

I rushed to the phone and dialed my brother's phone number. My niece picked up the phone.

"Hi Aunt Jean. My Daddy was expecting to pick you up at the airport today." She said, before I was able to get in a word.

"Well, It's a long story. I have been in the doctor's office and hospital all day." I explained to her.

"Oh no! Let me get my Daddy for you."

"Okay," I said.

I was really tired and it seemed like a long time before my brother came to the phone.

"Jean," he cheerfully said.

"I am as sick as a dog. If there is such a thing as being as sick as a dog," I told him.

"What's the problem?" He asked me.

Bloody Monday Fibroid Tumors....My Ordeal

"I have this awful pain in my right side. The pain is really bad at times. I have been in the doctor's office all day. The doctors took a lot of tests and they are not sure what is causing the pain, but they believe it is from the fibroid tumors. I am so sorry that I did not make it today." I told him.

I went on to explain to him about the problem. I must have really burned his ear. My brother is so sweet. He's the kind of person you can tell anything to. We have always had a wonderful relationship.

"Well my dear brother, I didn't want to get sick in Tennessee and have unfamiliar doctors taking care of me. I am so sorry," I sadly told him.

"Well your health comes first. We will have the meetings and email you the information. Is that okay?" He asked.

"Yes, that will be okay." I told him.

"Can you fax us the plans and the estimated costs?" He asked.

"I can do that. Listen, I hate to cut things short but I am really exhausted and I need to get some rest," I told him.

"Okay. Take care of yourself. We will be okay. I'll keep you informed with everything that is going on," he said.

I hung up the phone and told my daughter that I was going to bed. I couldn't rest. The pain was slight and I tossed and turned most of the night. It seemed that I could not get into a comfortable position. Finally morning came. I felt as if my whole body had been through the spin cycle in the washer machine. I didn't get out of bed. I decided to just lie there. I really did not have anything to do today. So, I slept for another four hours.

It was nice to be at home and just slum around. My daughter said she was hungry, so I go up and prepared breakfast for her and went back to bed. I just did not have the strength to get out of the bed. The pain was better and I did not have to take any pain killers, which for me was good. A few days later, my doctor called me with the test results.

"Jean, the test results are good. The blood count is normal," he said.

"Oh, that's good."

"We also took a look at the results of the ultrasound. You really have some large fibroids. We confirmed that there are two of them. They are about the size of two small oranges, and they may be causing the pain you are experiencing in your side." He explained.

"You think so?" I asked him.

"Yes, I do. But, everything looks okay. I'll need to send the ultrasound scans to your gynecologist. I'll need her fax number." He said.

"Okay, I'll get it and call you back." I told him.

I told the doctor goodbye and told my daughter and husband that the tests were normal. I went on to tell them that the pain in my side was most likely caused by the fibroid tumors.

A few days later and the pain were gone. The doctor did not recommend any additional treatment for the pain, because he felt that the fibroid tumors were causing the problem. The doctor did advise me to seek treatment for the fibroid tumors. When the pain was totally gone, I returned to business as normal.

BLOODY MONDAY. On June 19th, my cycle appeared to be heavier than normal for the second day. We had one of our religious meetings on Mondays at 7:30 p.m. Because of the heavy bleeding I had already decided not to go. Instead I decided to take a bath, wash my hair and go to bed. Maybe this will make me feel better.

I had completed my bath and was washing my hair in the shower, when the bleeding became worst. The clotting was so excessive that the large clots clogged the bathtub drain. Blood was literally running from my body like water. The water from the shower was filling the bathtub with the bloody water swirling around my feet. I turned the shower off, and watched as the blood and clots went down the drain.

"Oh no! Oh no!" I said out loud to myself as I got out of the shower, and the blood continued to gush out of my body down my legs onto the floor. The two white towels I was using had turned red and were soaked with blood.

I felt faint as I sat down in the bathroom. My breathing was getting heavier. I felt hot and sweat was pouring off my face. At this point I knew I had lost too much blood. I stood up to go into the bedroom and had to hold onto the bathroom wall and sink. I couldn't stand up by myself. I was afraid of falling because I was so weak. I don't remember how I got dressed, but somehow I managed to get on some clothes and made my way to the chair in the bedroom.

I called out to my husband. When he walked into the room I told him. "Please call the doctor. I'm bleeding really heavy, and I am so weak."

At that moment, I began to feel sick to my stomach. Needless to say I could not make it back to the bathroom and up on the bedroom floor and wall.

"I'm sorry." I said to my husband as he looked at me in shock. I had never been this sick before.

"What's your doctor's number. You need to call the doctor." He told me.

"I'll call her." I told him.

I called the doctor and the answering service said that the doctor on call would call me back within the hour. She also advised me that if it was an emergency to go directly to the hospital. It seemed like an eternity before the doctor called me back, but it was really less than an hour.

"Ms Alexander, this is the Doctor Rain. What problems are you experiencing today?" She asked with concern.

"My period is on and I am bleeding quite heavy. The clots are very large," I told her.

"Do you feel faint or have you been vomiting?" She asked.

"Yea, I do feel faint, and I did vomit one time," I told her.

"It sounds like you have lost too much blood, and I think you feel that you have lost too much blood. Are you near a hospital?" She asked.

"Yes I am," I told her.

"I want you to go to the emergency room right now. They can check to see if you have lost too much blood. The hospital will let us know what the results are." She said.

"Okay." I said and told her what hospital I was going to.

I hung up the phone and began to get dressed to go to the hospital. As I was getting dressed, my husband was busy cleaning up the mess I had made on the floor and walls in the bedroom. I don't know who cleaned up the mess in the bathroom. I don't remember cleaning it up. I never asked and no one ever told me.

My youngest daughter decided to come to the hospital with us. It normally takes us about 15 minutes to get to the hospital. It seemed like hours. I felt myself getting weaker and weaker. We arrived at the hospital about 7:00 P.M.

"Why didn't you stay home with the other kids?" I asked my daughter.

She responded, "Well, I will just be worried about you and calling Daddy all the time, so I decided to come with you." She said.

"Oh, that's sweet." I replied.

For some strange reason I began to feel better, although I was still very weak. I signed in and took a seat in the waiting room. Finally the medical receptionist called my name and had me fill out the necessary paperwork. When the paperwork was completed, she then put the hospital tag on my arm. I went back to my seat. The bleeding appeared to be getting lighter. Just as I sat down the nurse called my name.

Bloody Monday Fibroid Tumors....My Ordeal

As the nurse took my vital signs, she asked me about the problems I was having.

"I am bleeding very heavy and I feel weak and faint. I am feeling a little better now."

"You may have lost too much blood." She told me.

"How many pads are you using in a one hour period?" She asked.

"About four or five," I replied.

"Oh, that's far too many," she said.

"Do you have fibroids?" she asked.

Yes, I do."

"Those things are known to cause heavy bleeding." She told me.

"You think so?" I asked.

"Yes, they can. We have had women coming in here looking like they are about to deliver, because their fibroids are so large." She said.

"They can get that big?"

"Yes they can. They can also cause the type of problem you are experiencing." She replied.

The nurse completed the tests and asked me my doctor's name. I gave her the doctor's name.

"Oh, she and I did clinical together. She's a very good doctor." She said.

"I think so. I have only seen her once, but I think she is very good." I said.

"Yes, she is. Okay we're finished. They will call you shortly." She said.

"Thank you." I told her.

I went to the bathroom and then back to the waiting room. The bleeding and clotting was less and I was feeling even better as long as I sat and did not move. It had been a long day. I tried to get comfortable in the waiting room, but could not. The waiting room was somewhat crowded, and noisy. The basketball finals were playing on every TV in the waiting room. Everyone was concentrating on the game. I don't care much about basketball and pulled out a magazine to read.

Sitting in the waiting room, waiting for the doctor seemed to be a lengthy process. I wonder did it really matter to them that I was bleeding and had lost a lot of blood?

"Ms. Alexander." The nurse called my name. "Come on back."

I got up and felt the blood rush from my body. Sitting still had fooled me. I also felt weak and faint as I walked to the exam room. The nurse gave me instructions to get totally undressed and she gave me a cloth gown to put on, not one of the paper ones.

"I need to go the bathroom." I told her.

"Go right around the corner, and then come back here." She said.

I managed to get to the bathroom and back to the room. When I arrived back to the room the nurse took my vital signs. She was chatting about something that I could not focus on or understand, because I felt so faint.

"Okay, I need to set some blood to do the lab tests," the nurse said.

At that moment the doctor came in and spoke to me. She also instructed the nurse to start an I.V. and to get a urine sample.

The nurse started the I.V. "Because you have lost a lot of blood, we need to get some fluid back into your body." She said.

"Okay." I said.

"You're not pregnant are you?" She asked.

"Oh no. I'm not pregnant." I told her.

The doctor came into the room again and began to ask questions.

"How long have you been bleeding heavy like this?" She asked.

"For about two years, but this is the first time I have bled this heavily." I told her.

"I'm going to examine you now." She said.

The doctor looked at the nurse and asked her about the urine sample. The nurse informed her that she had not taken it.

The doctor told the nurse. "The bleeding is so heavy that you will have to use a catheter to get the urine sample."

"Okay." The nurse said.

The doctor left the room and the nurse leaned over me and said, "Mrs. Alexander we are going to get a urine sample. This may burn a little, but it will take only a minute and it should be okay." She said.

"Okay." I said.

As the nurse put the catheter in place, I could feel the stinging. She advised me to relax and it would be easier. She was finished in no time.

"Okay we're finished." The doctor will be back in when the lab results are complete. In the meantime just try to relax," she said as she left the room.

My daughter came in the room and sat down. "So, how are you doing?" She asked.

"Okay, I guess. I am waiting on the lab tests to come back to see what's wrong." I told her.

"Okay." She looked at me and smiled slightly.

After that my daughter did not have much to say. She just sat there and looked at me. I could feel that she was worried. I was worried too. To ease the tension, I asked her to go and get her daddy for me. She left the room and a few minutes later her father came into the room.

"How are you feeling?" He asked.

"Well, I feel better. The test results are not back. I think they believe the fibroids are causing the problem." I told him.

"You are probably feeling better because of the IV. There's no place to sit in here," he said as he leaned on the bed.

"I'm just waiting on the doctor to come back with the results. I don't know if they are going to keep me or not. So, I am going to try and get some sleep. If you want you can wait in the waiting room, since there is only one chair in here. I'll send for you when the doctor comes back and give me the results." I told him.

"Okay." He said as he touched my shoulder and left the room.

My daughter decided to stay in the room. She was busy reading her book. It was about 2:00 A.M. and she really looked tired. I wished she had stayed at home with the other children. Before I could get that much needed wink of sleep the doctor walked into the room and leaned over my bed.

"Well, Ms. Alexander I have the lab results back. You have lost quite a bit of blood. Your count is down to 28. We didn't find anything else wrong from the blood tests. Your urine samples came back okay. The bladder infection you had is clear." She said.

"Oh, that's good." I managed a smile.

"I have talked to your gynecologist and we both agree that we need to get the bleeding to stop. The heavy bleeding appears to be caused by the fibroids. I am going to prescribe some hormone pills for you to take for the next ten days, to help stop the heavy bleeding. I am also going to give you some prenatal vitamins, iron pills, and something to control the nausea." She said as she began to write the subscriptions.

"Okay." I told her. I was so tired and sleepy; that anything she said would have been okay.

"Ms. Alexander, we can treat you here in the hospital, or you can go home. If you stay in the hospital it will be just until tomorrow." She explained.

"I think I would rather go home." I told her.

"Okay. But make sure you call your doctor's office to make an appointment to see her today, or as quickly as possible. After 10 days of taking these hormone pills your body is going to do some strange things." She said.

"I will." I told her.

"That's great. Hopefully we can avoid you having to come back to the hospital again for this problem. Take care of yourself." She smiled.

"The nurse will be back in to assist you, so you can go home." She told me and left the room.

A few minutes later the nurse came back into the room with more tubes and instruments.

"Okay, they are going to admit you." She said.

I instantly woke up out of my sluggish mood. "Oh no, the doctor just said I can go home." I told her.

"I have been ordered to give you blood and admit you for surgery." She said.

"You must have the wrong person. The doctor said I can go home." I said as I sat up on the bed.

"You are Janie Alexander, aren't you?" She said as she looked at the chart.
"No. I am not! I am Jean Alexander." I told her.

"Oh my goodness, I have the wrong chart!" She alarmingly said.

"Thank God!" I said.

"I am so sorry hon. Let me get the right chart. The lady across the hall has a problem similar to yours, and her doctor is giving her blood and admitting her for surgery." She explained.

"Wow, I am glad you caught that, because I have not agreed to take blood of any sort or have surgery." I told her.

"Okay, I'll get your chart and be right back. Oh, I am so sorry." She said.

My daughter was in the room the entire time, taking everything in but not saying much. I looked at her, and asked if she was okay. She assured me that she was fine.

The nurse came back into the room. "Okay I have the right chart! You are Jean Alexander. Right?" She asked.

"Yes, you have the right chart now." I told her.

"Okay. I am going to increase the IV to drip a little faster so we can get all of this into you before you go home." She said.

There was only a small amount of fluid left in the IV bag, and I was hoping it would take only a few minutes to empty. It was odd, but I really felt better. I had been lying down for a while, so I wasn't sure about how heavy I was bleeding. Finally, the IV bag emptied. The nurse was busy filling out the paperwork to release me.

My daughter looked at me and said, "The bag is empty. I'll take those tubes out of your hand."

"You can't do that. You don't even know how to do it." I laughed at her.

"Yes I do. I saw it on one of those medical shows on TV." She said.

The nurse turned around and looked at her and started to laugh. "Hon, this emergency room is nothing like the ones you see on TV. This is the real life." She said jokingly.

"Have you ever dated a doctor?" I asked her.

She turned and looked at me and smiled. "I have, but it's nothing like TV. You don't have time to date while you are on duty. You're just too busy."

She lifted my hand and said, "Okay, let me have your hand to take out the IV."

I felt a slight burning sensation as she pulled the needle from my hand.

"Okay Mrs. Alexander, you can get up and get dressed. You're free to go," she said.

"Oh good." I replied.

She put two sheets of paper in my hand. "First let me give you these instructions on what you need to do when you get home. Make sure you call your doctor today to make an appointment to see her as soon as possible. Okay?"

"I'll make the appointment as soon as her office opens." I told her.

The nurse took a few more minutes to explain the instructions on the two sheet of paper to me. She again advised me to call my doctor as soon as possible.

"Okay hon., take care of yourself." She said to me and then looked at my daughter and said. "I'll see you sweetie."

My daughter looked at the nurse smiling and said. "Okay."

"Thanks for everything." I told her as she walked out of the door.

I looked at my daughter and asked her if she could leave the room, while I got dressed to go home. I asked her to tell her Daddy that I would be ready to go in about ten minutes and I would come out to the waiting room when I was ready.

I got off the exam table. I felt a small rush of blood coming from my body, but it was nothing compared to what it was when

I came to the hospital. I got dressed, combed my hair and went to the waiting room where my daughter was waiting for me. My husband had gone to get the car. Just as I got ready to sit down he pulled up in front of the emergency room. He came into the hospital and helped me to the car.

He had a look of concern on his face, "Are you feeling better?"

"Yea, I'm okay. I am still a little weak, but other than that I am okay." I replied.

Bloody Monday Fibroid Tumors....My Ordeal

As we drove home, I laid my head back on the car seat and tried to sleep. It seemed as though I could feel every bump in the road. The trip home seemed like an eternity.

"Do you need your prescription filled now, or do you need it later on today?" My husband asked.

I looked at him. "It's 3:00 A.M. in the morning. I think we can wait until later in the morning. I'm okay for now."

As we neared home my husband said he was hungry, and we stopped at one of the all night diners to get food. My daughter had remained very quiet on the ride home, but now she perched up when food was mentioned. She told her Daddy what she wanted. I didn't order anything. My husband went inside to order the food.

My daughter and I were waiting in the car for him to come back with the food. When you're sick even the slightest wait seems like eternality. I watched through the car window as the waiters cleaned the tables and kept peeping at us in the car. Maybe he thinks we are going to rob them. Why is it taking them so long to fix the food? I was really beginning to feel tired and sleepy. We were only a couple of miles away from home. I just wanted to feel the comfort of my own bed.

Finally my husband came back to the car with the food. Just smelling it made me sick. When we got home my husband and daughter ate and I went to bed. Ah... it was good to be home. It was so good to be home, and I was very thankful that I did not have to stay in the hospital.

Later on that day we got the prescription filled, and I made an appointment with the doctor for the next day at 9:00 A.M. I had begun to bleed heavy again. I took the medication the doctor prescribed and went back to bed. I stayed in bed most of the day, and when I was not in the bed I was sitting in the chair in my bedroom near the bathroom. I had never been this sick before. I called work and requested the assistant to change my vacation to sick time. I reflected back on the history of my menstrual cycle and how it had changed over the years.

Bloody Monday Fibroid Tumors....My Ordeal

I will never forget the first time my period came. I was nine years old. I come from a large family of four brothers and eight sisters. It was the summer of 1963, a nice warm day. My whole family was playing baseball. I played in the outfield because I was a good runner when the ball was hit to my area. It was time for our team to bat. My underpants felt wet. It was hot and I thought it was just sweat. Well, at nine years old you don't pay much attention to these things.

Finally, it was my time at the bat. We could win the game. There was no one on base, and I did from time to time hit home runs. I am a left-hand batter, and as the ball came across the plate, I hit it as hard as I could. I hit a home run! I hesitated before I began to run to first base, to see if my older brother would catch the ball. He didn't catch the ball and I ran as fast as my little legs could carry me. My brother got the ball and threw it to the pitcher. I was approaching home plate as I watched the pitcher throw the ball to the back catcher.

My mother was on our team. My sisters and mother were screaming. "Run, Run!"

Somehow I got some extra strength and slid into home plate at the same time the catcher caught the ball.

My mother yelled, "Safe!" No one dared dispute her call.

My team was jumping and screaming, we had won the game. Through all the excitement I felt my underpants getting wetter. I decided to take a look. I went into my mother's room and looked. To my horror, there was blood in my underpants. I must have hurt myself when I slid into home plate. I reasoned. I got one of my baby brother's socks and soaked it with antiseptic and put it between my legs.

I began to scream, because the antiseptic was burning. I didn't know that one of my older sisters was looking at me. She began to laugh.

"You've got your period," she laughed as she gave me a wet towel to wipe off the antiseptic.

"What's that?" I asked.

"Here put this on and let's go for a walk and I will tell you," she said.

"Put it where?" I asked.

"In your underpants stupid! It will keep you from messing up your shorts," she said.

In those days, mothers didn't talk much about the changes a young girl went through. They just let it sort of happen, gave you the necessary items to use and hoped you learned from there.

My sister and I took a long walk through the cotton fields and we finally stopped by a pond filled with lots of frogs. She told me all about the menstrual cycle and how many days it would last, what to use and how to keep myself clean. She also told me not to let any boys touch me because now I could have babies. After about thirty minutes of talking, the frogs were distracting me. I was playing with the baby frogs and was holding one in my hand when I heard my sister raise her voice.

"Don't even let a boy touch your finger! Because you can…. have lots of baby frogs!" She said.

I looked at her with wide eyes and hurriedly threw the frog in the pond. I took what she said seriously for years, and even told my friends at school that if a boy touched your finger you will have lots of baby frogs.

From that day forward, I had normal, painless cycles, every twenty-eight days until 1998. Beginning in 1998 I started to have heavier cycles every other month. The second day was always the heaviest and sometimes I would have to stay home from work. I had gradually grown from just the maxi thin pads to the overnight pads and the super plus tampons day and night.

I reflected on what the doctor had told me about having fibroid tumors. She didn't tell me what they were or how they looked? I wondered. I had received some Internet articles about fibroid tumors from friends, but I had not gone on the Internet to look up the information for myself.

I got the health books out again and looked up fibroids. I was eager to find out more information. The Internet had hundreds of sites, and I found more than enough information about fibroid tumors. I compared the information in the books with the information on the Internet. The information about fibroids was beginning to make more sense. I was even able to find actual pictures of the tumor, which cleared my mind, about how my tumor may actually looks.

The books and the information from the Internet explained that fibroids are benign growth, and they are hardly ever cancerous. It is amazing that black women have fibroids more frequently than women of other races. No one really knows what cause fibroids, but it is believed that the level of estrogen in the body contributes to the growth of fibroids. Some doctors believe fibroid tumors are the result of toxins that build up in the body resulting in the development of fibroids in the uterus.

The symptoms of fibroids may be none regardless of the size or they may cause painful menstruation, anemic, fatigue bladder infection, and heavy bleeding. I was experiencing all of these symptoms. The pain was not so bad unless the blood clots were large. I had constant bladder infections and I drank cranberry juice almost daily to help control the problem. The anemia is the worst of all. I am tired most of the time after my cycle. My blood count has been low for so long that I don't think I know how it feels to have energy for any length of time.

The health books went on to explain about the different options a woman had to help with the problem. The standard treatment for years was to give a woman a hysterectomy when the fibroids became a certain size. The myomectomy procedure removes only the fibroids and does not remove the uterus. There is also another procedure called myoma coagulation that cuts off the blood supply to the fibroid, causing it to shrink. Still another procedure called hysteroscopy may be used to diagnose the condition of the fibroids, but it can also be used to remove the fibroids and can be performed in the doctor's office or the hospital.

Then I read about the coffee. The book said it had found that most women who have fibroids consume large amounts of coffee. Well that hit home. I love coffee! I only drank it in the morning. I know I drank at least four cups a day. If I am at home and make a 12 cups pot of coffee, I will drink the full pot. I just liked the way it tastes, when I added the sugar and cream. This is something I will have to cut back on or cut out altogether. This is not going to be easy for me.

Exercise was highly recommended to reduce the excess estrogen in the body. Most of the health books recommended that you get as close to your idea body weight as possible. Well, I was no where near my idea weight. I knew my weight could be causing some of the problems. I was doing some walking, and I had lost a few pounds. Losing the weight will be hard to do. I have been overweight for so many years. I would have to fight my body, my mind and my soul to change these habits!

The diet recommended was almost a complete vegetarian diet. The diet consists of lots of fruits and vegetables, legumes, some fish and any other meat that are free-range and grain feed in very small amounts. Where will I find that kind of meat? I heard talk of a health food store in the downtown area that sells this kind of meat, but I had never been to the store. My family and I eat meat everyday, and I had it for lunch too. This will be another thing that will be hard to cut back on.

The information went on to explain the nutrients and some herbs that may help to relieve the symptoms of fibroids and control heavy bleeding. Some of the nutrients recommended were Kelp, Primrose Oil, Vitamin E, Vitamin A, Vitamin C, B Complex vitamins, Zinc, L-lysine, a multiple vitamin daily and iron if needed. Each book gave a variation of nutrients to take.

That night I slept okay, and the next morning I prepared to go to the doctor. My husband stayed off from work to take me. I didn't trust myself driving. I was feeling better, but I was still weak.

When we entered the doctor's office and I signed in. My husband began to chat with a co-worker that he recognized. I just sat and waited for the nurse to call me.

"Mrs. Alexander?" The nurse called.

I got up and the nurse instructed me to follow her to the lab. I weighed in and the Lab technician checked my blood count. My blood count was down to 18.

"What's the normal count?" I asked the lab technician.

"The normal count for the hematocrit is between 35 and 45." She explained.

"You don't use the old way for the blood count anymore? It use to be 12 to 15."

"It's just the one we decide to use. But any way would work. Okay, we're finished. Go to the waiting room to your right and the nurse will call you soon." She said.

I went to the waiting room, after I stopped by the bathroom. The hormone pills appeared to be working. The bleeding had slowed. It was unthinkable that all of this was happening to me. As I sat in the waiting room, I began to read the book I brought with me. Just as I settled into reading the book, a young pregnant girl called me to come with her.

"Hi my name is Joan, okay, let's go into the exam room. You were in the hospital last night?" The doctor asked.

"Yes I was. I had heavy bleeding and I lost a lot of blood."

"Your chart says that you have fibroids and it is very possible that they are causing the problem. Get undressed from the waist down and put this paper sheet around you. I need to examine you. I'll be back in a minute." She said.

I looked at her and thought, she looks too young to be a doctor. When she left the room I took off my clothes, and sat on the table. A few minutes later, what I thought was the pregnant doctor came back into the room.

As she examined me she said. "You are still bleeding too much, even with the medication the hospital gave you.

"I know, but it is not as bad as it was last night."

"We need to get this bleeding stopped. We can give you a hormone shot to stop the bleeding," she said.

"What type of hormone shot?" I asked her.

"Oh, it's a hormone shot to reduce the estrogen in your body and stop the bleeding. We can give it to you today if you want. I can give you a prescription to have it filled downstairs and you can bring it back up here and we will give it to you," she explained.

"I need more information on this hormone shot. Give me the prescription, and I'll think about it."

"Okay, get dressed and I'll come back and get you." She told me and left the room.

As I got off the table, blood gushed out on the table, the footstool and the floor. Tears welled up in my eyes as I looked at the blood on the floor. I quickly got dressed took the sheet and towels and soap from the sink to clean up the mess.

I was puzzled that I was offered medication without the doctor explaining to me what it was, and what the side effects may be. This was not my regular doctor. I had seen my regular doctor when I was at the doctor's office the first time, and this was someone different.

The young pregnant doctor came back into the exam room and we went down to her office. At this point she began to explain the hormone shot to me. The only explanation she gave me was pamphlets to read about the hormone shot, and the side effects. She then gave me sample iron pills and a prescription for the hormone shot.

"Why can't I continue to take the pills, I received at the hospital instead of the hormone shot?" I asked her.

"We can't continue to give you the pills, because of your age. You are 46 and you are at a higher risk for a heart attack if you continue on the pills. The shot would be better for you," she explained.

"I am still taking the pills the doctor gave me at the hospital, and I don't want to take the shot too. Can I wait until I finish the pills and read these pamphlets before I make my decision?" I asked her.

She looked at me with concern. "Yes you can do that, but you can't afford to lose this much blood next month. If you have to go back into the hospital, and your blood count drops below 16, you will be at the point where we will have to give you a blood transfusion." She explained.

"I am not going to take blood under any circumstances, because of my religious belief," I told her.

"Okay then that is an even stronger reason to take the hormone shot, because you won't take blood. You could actually die if you lost too much blood when your cycle comes next month," she explained.

"Listen, I have a few more days before I am completed with the pills I got from the hospital. I have the subscription and when I make up my mind I will fill it, give you a call and then you can give me the shot." I told her.

"Okay. I am just concerned about you. Take care of yourself and eat liver to help build your blood back up." She said.

"I will. Right now I am not comfortable with taking the shot. I want to read these pamphlets you gave me first." I thanked her for the information and went to the waiting room to pay my co-pay. I made an appointment to have my blood count checked the next week. I went back to the main waiting room to get my husband, so we could go home.

In the car, I read the pamphlets for the three-month hormone shot. It explained why it was used for fibroids and how the ovaries are put in a resting state to prevent a monthly cycle. As I continued to read I found that this was the same shot used for birth control.

The side affects was something that I was concerned about. The Hormone shot could cause

- Hair Loss
- Lost of sexual desires
- Irregular bleeding
- Menstruation stopping
- Weight gain
- Nervousness
- Dizziness
- Stomach ache
- Headache
- Fatigue
- Mineral loss in the bones
- and a host of other side effects

I then read the other pamphlet about a much stronger hormone shot. This shot actually shuts down the ovaries to prevent a monthly cycle. Again I looked at the side affects. They were much the same as the first one. The more I read the more I was against taking the hormone shot. When we got home I talked to my husband about the shot and explained the side affects to him.

He patiently listened to me. "It's up to you if you want to take the shot. You do want to consider what would happen if you didn't take it," he said.

When we got home, I went to my favorite reading spot, the bathroom and read the pamphlets over and over again. Somehow this was a harder decision than I had imagined. I reasoned with myself that the side affects didn't happen to everyone. These are just side affects listed that different women had experienced.

The next week I went back to work. Everyone there was concerned about how I was doing.

I went to lunch with one of my co-workers. "I heard you were sick," she said.

"Yes. I went on vacation and got sick. It was a scare for me. I am really glad to be back at work," I told her.

"I'm glad to see you back. I was worried about you. Are you okay?" She asked.

"Well, I am not totally okay." I told her and explained what had happened.

"The doctor wants to give me this hormone shot to control the bleeding. I really don't want to take it. I've discussed it with my husband, and he said it was up to me," I told her.

I noticed that she had a worried look on her face.

"What's wrong?" I asked.

"All the years I have known you, I have never told you what to do. But, this time I am telling you to take the shot. I am concerned about you," she said.

"I don't know about this shot. I have read the pamphlets, and the side affects are awful. I really don't want to take the shot." I told her.

"Do you have much of a choice? What if you start to bleed heavy again, then what?" She asked.

"I am really scared. I am really scared. I just don't have enough information about this shot." I told her.

"Okay, do what's best for you," she said. I could sense that she had given up on convincing me to take the shot.

After lunch we went back to work. I thought about what my husband and my co-worker had said about what could happen if I did not take the shot. I think it was at that moment that I reluctantly made up my mind to take the shot, after I finished taking the hormone pills from the hospital. I really did not want to get into a situation where the loss of blood could threaten my life. The situation was in my control, at least for now.

There is one thing that continued to puzzle me. I still did not feel that I was getting enough information from my doctor about my condition and the recommended treatment. No one in the doctor's office had explained anything to me about fibroids. The doctor had not explained to me anything about diet, vitamins, or exercise to help my condition. I felt that something was missing. A doctor should be concerned about your whole well being and not just the medical side of you.

Everything was pretty much back to normal. I was still a little weak and my skin was pale because my blood count was still low. The following week, I went back to the doctor to get my blood count. It was coming back up. It registered at 24. While at the doctor's office, the young pregnant doctor talked to me again and asked me about the hormone shot. I assured her that I would let her know when I had the prescription filled and would call to make an appointment to take the shot. I went to the check out desk and made an appointment to return in a week to have my blood count checked again.

I asked the receptionist. "What is the young pregnant doctor's name?"

"Honey, that's not a doctor. That's a midwife." She told me.

"A Midwife?" I said shocked.

"Yes. She helps out your doctor. When she sees you she consults with the doctor about your condition before making a recommendation," she said.

"Oh, is that the reason I have not seen my regular doctor?" I asked.

To me something was not right. "Do I have to pay the co-pay? I just had labs done and didn't see the doctor."

"Yes, you will have to pay. You did consult with someone, so a co-pay is due today," she said.

"Oh, you mean the midwife?" I asked.

"Yes." She said.

"I am used to seeing a doctor, when I come to the doctor's office, and not a midwife. It doesn't seem fair to make a co-payment for a midwife. I'm not pregnant. I need to make an appointment with the doctor for next week." I told her.

From that point forward it was an endless number of office visits. They were all to check my blood count and to check the amount of bleeding. Not one of those visits did I see a doctor. I saw the lab technicians, the midwife, the nurse, but never the doctor.

After I completed taking the hormone pills, the bleeding stopped. It was about eleven days after I came from the hospital. What a good feeling not to bleed, I felt so good! I wanted to shout to the world that I was not bleeding! But, silently, I only told my husband, family and a few close friends.

I was still pondering over whether I should take the hormone shot. I talked to friends and family again to reassure myself. The decision was split among family members. Some of them advised me to take the shot, others advised me not to take the shot.

That weekend my family and I went on a picnic at one of the local park with friends. I met one of my best friends there.

We began talking and I told her. “I’ve been sick.”

“What’s wrong?”

I hesitated as we walked down the hill. “I have these two huge fibroids and they are causing me to bleed heavily at times.”

“I have the same problem, but I am doing something to help control the bleeding.” She told me.

“What are you doing?”

“I am taking vitamins and herbs and it helps with the heavy bleeding.” She told me.

“I am coming over to your house so we can further discuss this.” I told her.

“Okay.”

Bloody Monday Fibroid Tumors....My Ordeal

After the picnic was over I went home and could not wait to go to my friend's house. For the first time I felt as if I had an option to help with my problem. I still had not taken the hormone shot and according to my doctor, ah, the midwife, my time was running out.

The next week my friend and I got together at her house. She pulled out her many health books. We began to look at some of the things that are recommended for fibroids. We went over the causes of fibroids, what could be done to control excessive bleeding and what vitamins and herbs to take to help the problem. What I liked best about reading the health books were the clear instructions on how to fast and cleanse the body.

Some of the remedies mentioned took me back to my childhood. My mother use to give us certain teas to help with colds and other ailments we had. We also would take sitz baths for female ailments. Did these remedies really work? My friend and I both began to laugh when I read out loud about the cold and hot sitz baths.

"Jean." She said. "I think I like the sitz baths, but I don't think I can find a tub big enough to fit my butt."

We both laughed. "You're small. I told her. You can go to the hardware store and get a #3 tub. But I am with you on this one. I don't think I can move my butt from a cold tub of water to a hot tub of water. This seems like it would be not only tiring but a shock to my butt."

"But this is supposed to help shrink the fibroids. The hot water is supposed to force blood into the fibroids and the cold water forces blood out of the fibroids. Eventually this is supposed to shrink them." She said seriously.

"Where did you get this book?" I asked her.

"From the health food store. I'll make a copy of this page for you." She said.

"Oh no, I am going to buy it tomorrow. I need to get some vitamins, herbs and tea from the health store." I told her.

"I am really scared to take the hormone shot." I said taking on a more serious tone.

She looked at me lovingly. "Well, if you take the shot you will have 90 days to get your body healthier. You can get your body in better shape if you do have to have surgery to remove the fibroids. Think about it that way."

I felt so much better. My friend had made me feel better about taking the shot. She didn't tell me to take the shot. She gave me some possible benefits of taking the shot.

It was getting late and I had to leave. As we said goodbye at the door, I hugged her and thanked her for the information and the concern and love she had shown.

The next day I bought the book she had recommended. It was the best book I had ever read about natural treatments. I read everything that pertained to fibroids. Good tips were given on what to do to improve your health. The authors of the book never ruled out the possibility that surgery may still be needed to correct the problem. The advice they gave was excellent and was something that I felt I could follow.

I began to follow much of the advice the book gave and began to feel really good. I was feeling so good that I actually forgot about the shot the doctor had recommended. A few weeks later I went back to the doctor to check my blood count and it was normal.

When I left the doctor's office, I called my closest friend screaming. "My blood count is normal! My blood count is normal!"

"Good!

"I'm so excited! I'll talk to you later." I ended the conversation without saying goodbye.

A few days later, I looked at the prescription in my wallet. I thought about the advice my family and friends had given me. I thought about the possibility of heavy bleeding again. I read the brochure for the hormone shot again and again. Maybe I won't have any of these side effects. I convinced myself that it would not be too bad taking the shot. I made a firm commitment to take the shot.

I went to the drug store on July 2nd, and had the prescription filled. Although, I felt excellent, I knew that I could end up in the hospital again. I was afraid of having to go there again. I made an appointment on July 6th to have the nurse give me the shot. After I got to the doctor's office that morning, I went into the exam room with the nurse.

"Ms. Alexander, you're here to take hormone shot for fibroids to stop the bleeding right?"

"Yes, I am."

"Where will you like to take it? I usually like to give it in the hip. There's more meat back there and it won't hurt as bad," she said.

"That will be okay." I told her. I won't have any effects from this will I?"

"No. You'll be able to drive home. But let me tell you that these shots can actually cause bleeding. Some women have bled for months." She warned me.

"I'm glad you are telling me this now. I read the pamphlets. Am I taking the three month type hormone shot? I mean, I won't have to take this shot but once every three months right?" I asked her.

"No. To control fibroids, you will have to take this shot once a month. Didn't the doctor tell you this?" She asked.

"Once a month? This is supposed to last for three months. You're telling me that I will have to take this shot every month? That's a lot of hormones in my system!" I said with an expression of horror on my face.

"Yes I know but this is the way we treat the fibroids and hopefully stop the bleeding and possible shrink them." She said as she instructed me to pull my pants down enough to get to my right hip to give me the shot. I felt a small prick and it was over.

"Well, maybe I won't have the side effects. Thank you. Can I go now?" I asked her.

"Yes, you are all ready to go. I hope things work out okay for you. If you have any problems at all, give us a call." She said.

I went to the front desk and checked out, and went to work. I told a close friend at work that I had taken the shot.

"Oh no! I thought you were going to look into trying the natural way," she said.

"I was, but I am so afraid of bleeding again like that," I told her.

I went to my office and really did not think about the shot anymore. I was sure that it would work. Yet I had this nagging feeling deep in my mind that it would not work. That evening I called my oldest daughter and told her that I had taken the shot.

"Mommy! A girl I work with took that shot and she bled for months. Now, she doesn't have periods at all. She also gained a lot of weight! I hope this doesn't happen to you," she said.

"Well, I made the decision to take it. I am hoping that nothing like that happens to me. I feel fine and I just can't risk losing that much blood again." I said.

"Okay, let me know how things turn out." She said.

I had another week without spotting and then the spotting returned. Sometimes it was light requiring just a light liner. At other times it required heavier protection. The spotting and bleeding went on for twenty eight days. During that time I went to the doctor two times. I had my blood count checked, and it was okay, but I still did not see the doctor.

I saw the nurse, and the midwife, but not the doctor. When I told the nurse about the continuos bleeding. They were quick to tell me that the hormone shot was probably causing the bleeding.

Although, I was spotting and bleeding at times, my blood count had only dropped down to a count of 30.

I was becoming more and more concerned about not seeing the doctor and developing a doctor patient relationship. Since June 9th, I had made a total of five visits to the doctor's office and had seen the doctor only once.

I was also concerned that I had taken a shot that was supposed to control my bleeding and it had actually caused me to bleed for the last twenty eight days, and there was no way for me to reverse the effects of the shot. The shot also caused me to have what I considered severe emotional swings. I would cry at the drop of a hat. At the same time I could be very harsh. I had night sweats, and hot flashes. I didn't want to talk to anyone and pretty much stayed in my office for about a month.

During that twenty eight day period, I stayed at home a few days because the bleeding was heavier than normal. I had talked to my manager and told her that if I had to stay at home or leave work this would be the reason.

The worst thing for me was the commute to work. The construction of a new building near my work had begun, and parking was not available in the parking lot for employees. Because I didn't always know how much I would bleed, I decided not to take public transportation to work. I didn't want to be embarrassed if I should have an accident. This is why I drove to work, and hunted for a parking spot. I felt that it would be better for me to walk the short distance to my car and drive home if needed. My daughter also lived near my work, so if things got really bad I could always go to her apartment until things got better.

Bloody Monday Fibroid Tumors....My Ordeal

Many times when I could not go to work or had to leave work, I would call to let my manager know that "My body was not acting right." This was my code to my manager to let her know that the bleeding was bad.

One morning I called work to inform my manager that I would not be coming in. When my body was acting up, it was always better to work at home. I was so glad that I had that option from time to time. I could relax when needed and still finish up my assignments. It was also a good time to clear out my voice mail and call clients that I could not call, because we are always so busy at work.

The thing that bothered me most is the extra responsibility I had to put on the senior person in my area. He had to take on management responsibilities along with his normal work assignment. He constantly told me to take care of myself and that everything was okay at work. We have been working together for over ten years and I knew that I could depend on him totally, but I still felt guilty. I called him and told him that I would be back to work the next day, because I was feeling better.

The next morning, I was rambling through my closet for something to wear. I began to realize that my condition was changing my life style. I was slowly beginning to hate the colors I love most, black and navy blue. I had been wearing long black and navy blue skirts, dresses, and pants, for over a month. If I had an accident it would not show and I could at least make it back to my car without being noticed.

I wanted to wear something different. Something a little brighter than black. I pulled out a light purple suit. The skirt came to my knees it was one of my shorter suits. I also pulled out my favorite short blue suit. A light green suit, and a pink suit.

I smiled. All of these would really look great. I feel like wearing something different, but something inside was nagging at me.

"Wear something long and dark." Wear something long and dark." My conscience tugged at me.

I had worn all of my dark long clothes, and most of them were in the cleaners. I felt defeated. Then I looked in my youngest daughter's closets and found her red flower long dress. The dress was too big for her but it was a perfect fit for me, and it came down to my ankle.

"I think I will wear this one with my red jacket." I knew she wouldn't mind me wearing it, because I had worn the dress once before.

When I arrived at work John looked at me and said "Jean, how are you doing?"

"I'm okay. A little weak, but I'm here," I told him.

You don't look well. You are always telling us to take care of ourselves and you even send us home when we have just a little cold. So, I am telling you to go home and take care of yourself," he said.

"I'm okay. I do need you to continue to help me out. I am going to be in my office most of the day catching up and completing these reports." I told him.

"Okay. Now you know that we can handle things if you need to stay out longer," he said.

"I know. I am a little weak, but really I can make it." We hugged and I was thankful that I had such a wonderful and loving team.

I had made it through the day. It was about 5:00 P.M. and I was preparing to go home. My team was also packing up to go home. I got up from my chair and felt this huge rush of blood. I called John and told him to tell Nini not to leave. I couldn't tell him why, but I needed her to take me to my daughter's apartment.

I got my bags and headed for the bathroom. As I passed the elevator, I felt the blood running down my legs. I began to walk faster toward the bathroom. Tears began to well up in my eyes. Just as I entered the bathroom, the blood was running down my legs onto my shoes and onto the floor.

"Oh no! Oh no!" I cried, as the tears began to run down my cheeks.

I noticed that no one was in the bathroom and I thanked God for that. Before I took care of myself I rushed and pulled napkins from the dispenser, wetted them and cleaned the blood from the floor. I didn't want anyone to come into the bathroom and be alarmed seeing blood on the floor.

Thank God I had worn the long red flowered dress. The dress was not soiled. I could not imagine what the results would have been if I had worn one of the shorter light colored suits. I cleaned up as much as I could. Just as I completed, one of the other managers from my department entered the bathroom.

"Jean are you okay?" She asked.

"Yeah. I guess I am. The hormone shot the doctor gave me is not working. I have been bleeding since I took the shot." I told her.

Nini entered the bathroom and asked. "Jean you need me to take you somewhere?"

"Yes I do. I can't walk to my car. I am bleeding pretty heavy. Could you take me to my daughter's apartment?"

"Yeah. Do you need me to bring the car around to pick you up?" She asked.

"No. I think I can walk to the parking garage." I told her.

Nini was in a company car and had the privileges of parking in the company's parking garage, which was a short walk from the building.

"Jean I am going to have to drop John off at his car will that be okay?" She asked.

"Yes, that will be okay." I said.

We got to the car and dropped John off at his car. Nini then dropped me off at my daughter's apartment.

"Thank you Nini. I really appreciate this." I told her.

"That's okay. I am beginning to have the same problem, and I know what you are going through. Take care of yourself." She said.

I went into my daughter's apartment and called my husband to come and get me. My husband arrived about an hour later.

"I am so glad you are here. I need to pick up my car. I think I can drive home," I told him.

"Are you okay? Do you need to go to the doctor?" He asked me with concern.

"No. I think I am going to be okay." I told him as I sat back in the car seat and closed my eyes.

"I didn't want to take that shot. I was afraid this would happen. I have been bleeding all month." I angrily told my husband without letting him get a word in.

My husband looked at me and said. "Maybe you should try something else."

I didn't respond to him and the trip to my car was a silent one. We made it to my car and I managed to drive home. I called work and left voice messages that I would not be in the next day.

The next day I was bleeding really heavy. I called and made an appointment with the doctor. I had been spotting and bleeding now for over 35 days. The doctor saw me and ordered a blood count. Finally I get to see the doctor. I was not very friendly or pleased that this was only my second time seeing the doctor in the last two months.

The doctor came in the room and I knew that she sensed my concerns and displeasure. " I see your blood count is down to 24. The hormone shot did not work."

"No it's not working and I have been bleeding for more than 30 days!" I told her.

"Well, you know that the hormone shot can cause bleeding," she said.

"I wish you had explained that to me before and not just give me a pamphlet. Bleeding continuously is worst than having a heavy period, letting your blood count go down and getting it over with until the next month." I told her.

She appeared to not hear what I said. "Jean, I want you to take another hormone shot. Sometimes the first one does not work, but the second one will stop the bleeding."

"Okay." I told her. At this point I would take anything to stop the bleeding.

The doctor looked at the nurse and told her to give me the second shot. I took the shot but had already made up my mind that I would be looking for another doctor. I was not pleased with the way the doctor was managing my health. Fibroids may be common to black women, but they were not common to my body.

Bloody Monday Fibroid Tumors....My Ordeal

It takes only a few minutes for doctors to explain what to expect from fibroids. I had asked questions, but the doctor seemed too busy to give me a few minutes of her time. I had received more information from the health books and the Internet than from my doctor.

I heard the doctor tell the nurse to schedule me for an endometrial procedure for the following month. She did not explain what this procedure was or how I should prepare for it. She did tell me that it could possibly tell her what was causing the bleeding.

I went to the check out desk and made the appointment to have the procedure done on September 1st. I left the doctor's office very displeased. I was also angry at myself for not following how I felt about taking the hormone shot. I made up my mind that I was not going to take another hormone shot. Taking the second shot did not stop the bleeding. On September 1st, I went back to the doctor for the endometrail procedure. The nurse prepared me for the procedure. To my surprise the doctor came into the examination room to do the procedure.

"I can't do this procedure. She is still bleeding." The doctor said to the nurse.

"If you had explained to me that I could not be bleeding when this procedure is done, I could have stayed at home. Do I have to pay for this?" I asked.

The doctor looked at me without answering and pulled my eyelid down. "Your blood count is still low. Are you taking your iron pills?"

"Yes, I am."

"I am thinking about having the operation to have the fibroids removed since nothing else is working." I told the doctor.

"You are? She asked. All of a sudden, the doctor appeared to be interested in talking to me.

"Well, we can take the fibroids out without removing the uterus. I will need a week's notice. Call this number and make an appointment when you are ready to schedule for surgery." She said as she wrote down the number and the name of the person to contact on a sticker pad and gave it to me.

I am sure the doctor sensed my dissatisfaction with the lack of information and what appeared to be a lack of concern for my health.

The doctor left the room and the nurse came in the room. "We don't have your ultrasound tests for the fibroids and we will need them before the operation is performed. Did your primary Doctor send them?"

"Yes, my primary doctor faxed them to you back in June. You're just noticing that they are not here?" I asked her.

"Let me check with the other nurse." She said as she left the room.

The nurse came back in the room and said. "We don't have them. Can you have your doctor fax them to us again?"

"Okay I will." I told her in what was now an irritated voice.

I got dressed and could not believe that I had put up with this doctor for such a long time.

As I checked out the doctor came to the checkout desk and said. “Don’t forget to take your iron pills and eat right.”

“I will.” I told her holding back my anger.

The rest of September was pretty much the same as August. Some days I would have moderate to heavy bleeding and other days it would only be light spotting.

On September 20th, I had a conference with one of our departments at the local colleges to explain the changes that our department was making to better serve their area. I will never forget that day. The bleeding stopped for one day!

I was so happy. Unfortunately I ate something that made me very sick. I could not enjoy the short period of not bleeding. I went home and stayed in bed for about two hours and then went back to work. Regardless of the small problem with an upset stomach, I still enjoyed the day without bleeding.

In September my first grandchild was born. I told my son that I would be there seven days after the baby was born. Like all other times my body was not acting right and I could not go. The bleeding was so heavy that I did not trust myself traveling.

Finally on October 15th I made plans and reservations to go to California. I took two weeks vacation. On October 20th, although still spotting I went to California to visit my son and his family. I was so excited and could not wait to see my grand-baby.

My son picked me up at the airport. I was so glad to see him. I had not seen him in over a year! We hugged and headed for his car. I looked in the car hoping that he had brought the baby.

“Where’s the baby?” I asked him.

“Oh she’s at home. I didn’t think we could all get in this car with your luggage.”

“Oh.” I said disappointed because he had not brought my daughter in law and the baby.

"You look good. Are you feeling okay?" He asked.

"Yes, I am feeling great. I am thinking about having the operation when I get back home. But, I have some concerns about my doctor," I told him.

We pulled up in front of the apartment and the conversation was cut short. I was excited about seeing the baby. I walked into the apartment and was introduced to my son's wife and his wife's sister. We hugged. Both my son's wife and her sister looked exactly the way they looked in the pictures my son had sent over the Internet.

Finally I got to see the baby. "Oh she is so beautiful!" I said as I cradled her in my arms.

My son began to take pictures. He took lots of pictures of the baby and me. The baby seemed to enjoy me holding her. I could not take my eyes off her.

"You all can do whatever you want to do. Just leave the baby with me." I told my son and his wife.

They laughed at me. "We have not been out since the baby was born. We may take you up on that and go out this weekend."

"Whatever you want to do." I said without looking up from the baby.

I instantly fell in love with this beautiful little person. For a moment I had forgotten about my condition and had focused all of my attention on her. Every part of her was beautiful!

I was thankful that God had answered my prayers. The first three days I was in California I did not have any spotting. Then on October 25th, I began to have some spotting. Again, I prayed to God for the spotting to stop. I was afraid that I would start to bleed and have to go to the hospital in California.

Although, I was not pleased with my doctor, I did not want to put my health in the hands of strangers. I was leaving on Tuesday and I prayed and prayed that the spotting would stop. Again, my prayers were answered. The spotting stopped. Although, I enjoyed my grand daughter and spent all of my time with her, I was eager to get home. I was eager, because I was afraid of my body not acting right. More and more my condition was beginning to put limits on my life.

Bloody Monday Fibroid Tumors....My Ordeal

After I returned home from California, I was feeling better. I was eating better, and had limited my coffee drinking to about two cups a month. This was the second month without the hormone shot. Even with the constant spotting this was a good month. It was always in my mind that the hormone shot I had taken was really causing the prolonged bleeding. I had found information on the Internet about how long the hormones stated in your system. Since I had actually taken a six months dose in two months, I had to wait three or more months for it to get out of my system. Then I reasoned that my body would go back to normal and I would have the seven or eight days period, that would be heavy for a few days. I would rather have this than to bleed continuously all the time.

My family and I spent October 28th and 29th in Alabama to attend a convention. Although I was spotting, I prayed that I would make it through the weekend. When we returned home a friend and I was talking about endometriosis and she mentioned her doctor and how good she was. I had already decided to change doctors, what could I lose by seeing her? I decided to make an appointment the following week to see the doctor. I called the doctor's office and made an appointment for November 22nd.

Despite constant spotting on November 8th, I started what seemed to be a normal cycle. At first the bleeding was light and eight days later I was still bleeding. On November 15th, the bleeding was very heavy and painful. I was afraid to go to work. I called work informing them that I would not be coming in. To my surprise the heavy bleeding stopped after about an hour. I was still afraid to go to work the next day because I could never predict when the bleeding would be heavy.

A friend called me at home. "Jean how about lunch today."

"Oh, I can't." I said

"Your body acting up?"

"Yes! How did you know?" I asked

"I just know. I guess you are staying at home because you don't want to have an accident," she laughed.

I laughed with her. "I guess you are right about that. Actually it's not that bad. It just scares me to think of what would happen if I had gone to work today."

"Okay Jean. Maybe we can get together next week?" She asked.

"Okay. That will be great." I said, and got back in the bed.

Bloody Monday Fibroid Tumors....My Ordeal

I had not been bleeding or spotting for a few days and on November 22nd, I went to the gynecologist recommended to me by my friend. As I entered the office, the waiting room seemed a little junky. There were payment notices and newspaper articles posted all over the walls.

I filled out the necessary paperwork and waited to see the doctor. I was feeling a little scared, because I had some spotting the night before and I had hoped to be free of bleeding when I saw the doctor. As I waited, I decided I might as well read the newspaper articles about alternative medicine and nutrition posted on the wall. This may be a good doctor after all. The articles on the wall about alternative medicine and nutrition were exactly what I was looking for. Just as I was getting through the second article, the nurse called me.

I followed the nurse to the lab, and she took my weight and blood pressure. She then took me to an examination room. I got undressed and put on the paper gown. I had resolved not to complain about the paper gown anymore. After about ten minutes the doctor walked in. I was startled to see how unconventional she was. She had a wrap on her head about twelve inches tall, and very colorful.

"Hi, Mrs. Alexander. You are here to see me about the fibroid tumors you have?" She asked.

"Yes, I am." I said.

"Okay, let's examine you." She said.

"You have some pretty large fibroids. About fourteen to sixteen weeks." She said.

"Yes, I know."

The doctor completed the exam and asked me to come to her office. When I got to her office we talked about some things that can be done about fibroids. She mentioned the order in which she would treat me, first by using a low estrogen birth control pill. The next steps would be myomectomy or a hysterectomy.

“What about Uterine Artery Embolization procedure?” I asked.

She hesitated before speaking. “Oh yes, that is a new procedure and you can have that done over at the hospital.”

“I read about it in the paper, and it is something that I may be interested in having done.” I said.

“Well, you will have to make arrangements with the hospital to have the procedure done.” She told me.

“You don’t do the procedure?” I asked.

“No. The Interventional Radiologist at the hospital will do it.” She said and changed the subject to focus on the sheet of paper she placed in my hand.

Before I could speak again, she said. “I want you to consider trying this for your bleeding. You can buy the book if you want. It may help with your problem. You can pick up the book at any bookstore.”

I looked at the information and it basically recommended what the other health books had. Change your diet take certain vitamins and eliminate trans-fatty acids from the diet. We talked about the book and I told her that I might buy it.

Bloody Monday Fibroid Tumors....My Ordeal

"Okay Mrs. Alexander, I will see you in one year. Try to get your weight down, this will help with the estrogen level in your body. Oh, I need to get a blood count. Well maybe not today."

I left out of her office dazed. She didn't order a blood count, and she wanted to see me a year from now. She did not even mention that if I had problems to call the office.

I was impressed with the doctor and her approach to natural and conventional medicine, but I was disappointed with her approach to handling my problem. I wondered, are fibroids so common that they are not seen as a serious problem for women?

December 3rd, sad news came about my sister's husband death. The funeral activities would begin on Saturday, with the burial on morning. I arranged to take Friday and Monday off from work to go to the funeral in St. Louis, Mo. I called a few airlines to see if I could get some good ticket prices, but at such late notice I was not able to.

"Well, I can't get a good fare, so I guess we should drive." I told my husband.

"Okay. I guess we can rent a car and leave Friday morning." He said.

"Okay, but only if my body is acting right," I told him.

On December 4th, my period started. I had been taking kelp and parsley daily, increasing it during heavy bleeding and it appeared to be working. Thursday night the bleeding was very heavy. Sadness filled my heart. I knew that I would not be going to St. Louis for the funeral.

"Jean are you still going?" My husband asked.

"It looks like I won't be going. I'm bleeding too heavy." I said as I felt the tears burning in my eyes. "I'll call my sister tomorrow and let her know why I can't make it."

My condition had began to interfere, it appeared with each important event occurring in my life. Friday morning was just as I expected it to be. Throughout the day the bleeding was extremely heavy, each cramp producing clots the size of a small orange. I knew that the stress I was feeling was contributing to the heavy bleeding. I didn't want to go back to the hospital, so I go up and took my vitamins, iron pills with extra kelp and parsley.

I was afraid that I might be losing too much blood. I kept looking under my lower eyelids to see if they were pink or red. If they were red it meant that my blood count was okay. If they were pink or white it was an indication that my blood count was getting low. When I looked under my lower eyelid, to my surprise they were still red. At the end of the day I looked under my eyelid again and they were light pink. This was an indication that my blood count was falling.

All day I ignored the fact that I was getting weak and tired. I did not want to go to the hospital again. I did not want to take hormones to stop the bleeding. I prayed and prayed to God not to stop the bleeding, but to make it bearable for me and to make the blood flow moderate. I also prayed that I would not feel so stressed. I had read that stress could also cause the menstrual flow to be abnormal.

I gathered up enough strength to prepare dinner and decided to call my sister before I went to bed. When I called my sister, I did not expect her to pick up the phone. I explained to her that I was sick and would not be able to make it to the funeral. We had a long conversation about the last days of her husband's life. Sadness filled my heart because I could not be there to comfort her when she needed it the most.

I spent most of Saturday just sitting around the house. I was getting weaker and weaker. I knew that my blood count was getting lower, because I could feel my joints. I could feel all of the joints in my fingers, elbows, hips, and knees. Anywhere there were bones connected together, I could feel them. It's hard to explain how the joints feel. They are not stiff. It is more like soreness, but your body is not really sore.

I didn't get out of bed that day because my breathing was heavier and I felt I would be better off if I got lots of rest. I continued to take my vitamins, iron, kelp and parsley. Sunday was much better. The bleeding was much lighter, and although weak I felt much better. I was scheduled to return to work the following Monday. I didn't have the strength to get out of bed. I sat up in bed and wondered when would this all end.

Bloody Monday Fibroid Tumors....My Ordeal

I had to get my life back to some sort of normalcy. I got out of the bed and was determined to put on clothes and get out of the house. I took a shower, and washed my hair. My cell phone was ringing and it showed a number that I didn't recognize so I didn't answer it. I was toweling off my hair, and wondered who was calling me. I tried to call the number back, but didn't get an answer.

"Well, whoever called, left a message." I said to myself as I listened to the message.

"Jean, this is James. Your husband is on the way to the hospital. Please give me a call." The message said.

Alarmed, I called my husband's work and got more information. I came into the kitchen where my son and daughter was sitting and told them their father was in the hospital and sent them to the hospital ahead of me.

I was concerned about driving to the hospital. I had not driven in a few days. I got in the car and everything was okay, until I got on the expressway. The car felt like it weighed ten tons and the steering wheel felt like I was turning a block of bricks. I did not realize that I was so weak. I decided to drive slower, because controlling the car was a task. The trip to the hospital was a long one. Finally, I saw the hospital exit. I looked for a parking space near the hospital. I didn't want to park too far from the hospital, because I was weak and didn't want to do too much walking. Finally, I found a parking space in front of the hospital.

I entered the emergency room and gave the receptionist my husband's name. She directed me to his room. When I entered the room, I saw that my husband was asleep. I sat on the stool beside his bed and rested my head against the hospital wall for support because I was so weak.

After a while, my husband woke up. I stood up and touched his arm. "Sweetie, how are you? I need to go to the bathroom. You rest and I'll be right back."

"I'm okay and I am not going anywhere." He looked at me and smiled.

There is only one bathroom to use in the emergency room. As I entered the bathroom, my period was flowing like water. I felt so helpless, because I was so weak. I became very angry, as I looked at the blood on the floor and on my legs. I began to cry silent tears.

"I need to be in the hospital. I need to be in the hospital. Why is this happening to me?" I said out loud.

I was praying that my husband would not be at the hospital long. I wanted to be there for him, but I felt so helpless. I had always been strong and now I was so weak that even sitting at the hospital was draining me of the little strength I had left.

I looked at the mess I had made in the bathroom and realized that being angry would not help my situation. I couldn't give my condition back. I couldn't solve the bleeding problem by myself. I couldn't even walk away from my condition. Strength or no strength I had to be strong for my husband. He needed me to be there for him.

I began cleaning up the mess I made on the floor. Just as I finished taking care of myself and cleaned up everything, the doorknob on the bathroom door began to rattle. Whoever wanted to get in kept rattling the doorknob. Finally the person began to knock on the door.

"Okay. Okay. I'm coming out." I yelled at the door as I looked around the bathroom to make sure that everything was clean, before I opened the door.

"Oh, I am so sorry," the lady said. "The nurse told me to knock."

"That's okay. It's a shame that there is only one bathroom to use in here." I said as I walked past her and headed back to my husband's room. Finally after another three hours, my husband was released from the hospital and we went home.

On December 19th, the spotting stopped. I was so excited! I didn't tell anyone because so many times before, I thought the spotting had stopped, only to be disappointed. The next day I was still spot free!

I called my closest friend Janice, very excited. "The spotting stopped! The spotting stopped! I haven't spotted since Tuesday!" I screamed.

I heard Janice laugh out loud.

"I know this is not exciting conversation for you and it can't be the most interesting thing to talk about, but I can breathe down there!" I said excitingly.

"I'm happy for you!" She Said.

"Okay. I won't hold you any longer. Goodbye."

I hung up the phone and laughed out loud and danced around the room. Although I was excited, I still could not believe that I had been spot free for almost two days. Being spot free did not last for long. On December 24, the bleeding began again. I told my husband about it and told him that there were some things I wanted to get done. I knew that the bleeding would eventually get heavy and I would not be able to go anywhere. I tried to do everything in that one day. We went out to eat dinner, to the bookstore and the mall. It was a busy but good day.

On, New Year's day, I was having horrible cramps. I told my husband that it was menstrual cramps. He helped me into bed, and put the heating pad on my stomach. I took pain medicine to ease the pain. I was up and down all night and very restless.

To my surprise and pleasure it was not menstrual cramps. I had the flu! Can you imagine being grateful that you had the flu? For the next few days I ran a high fever and stayed in bed. The spotting was so light that protection was not even needed. What a relief, I couldn't imagine having the flu and bleeding heavy at the same time.

A few days later, I was feeling better from the flu. The spotting was getting heavier and I began to pass large blood clots again. It was so bad. I sat in the chair in my bedroom to be closer to the bathroom. I sat in that chair Friday, Saturday and Sunday both day and night. I was up and down from the chair to the bathroom, every thirty minutes. I was very exhausted, as weakness gripped my body.

It is strange, but I felt something different happening to me. It was not my physical condition. It was fear. I was becoming afraid to go to work or to any other social functions when I was bleeding. Fear was gripping me. My condition was controlling not only how I dressed, but also my every action.

"What am I going to do?" I asked myself. My condition was not getting any better. My life is becoming consumed by my condition. I was wearing only black and navy clothing all the time. Once a very confident and active person, I was becoming glued to my house.

I had become a well equipped drugstore for feminine products. I had a good stock in my desk drawer at work, my brief case and my purse. My car carried a full supply of protection of any kind you can imagine. The glove compartment and armrest in my car was stuffed with feminine items. The book bag in the trunk of my car was overstuffed with tampons. I had feminine items in my dresser drawers, stuffed under the bathroom sink and under my bed.

Bloody Monday Fibroid Tumors....My Ordeal

On January 10th, I was walking from the parking lot to my office building. As I stood at the red light, I felt a warm rush of blood. I had been bleeding for about eighteen days. I prayed that I would make it to the building as I felt another large rush of blood leave my body. It seemed like an eternity before the light turned red and the walk sign came on. I rushed across the street entered the building and dashed for the bathroom. Tears flowed down my face as the large clots pushed out of my body.

"I can't continue with this. I can't do this anymore." I said under my breath.

Somehow, I managed to get myself together and at that moment I made up my mind to take time off from work, and take care of my problem. I went to my office, deposited my bag and purse. I walked into my manager's assistant office and asked if I could see her when she came in.

"What time do you want? Are you okay?" She asked as she looked up at me with deep concern in her eyes.

"No, I'm not okay." I told her.

"Okay, I understand. You can see her when she gets here, around 9:00 A.M.," she said.

Before the words were out of the assistant's mouth, the manager walked up. The assistant told her that I wanted to see her right away.

"Come on in." She said in a cheerful voice.

"Thanks for seeing me on such short notice. Well, you know about my condition and it is not getting any better." I told her.

"Yes, I do. How is it going?" She asked.

"Not too good. I am weak most of the time and I just cannot go on like this. I am here because I need to take time off to build up my body and decide what I am going to do about these fibroid tumors." I told her.

"That's okay with me. You have to take care of yourself. If you don't you won't be able to take care of your family or your work." She said in a caring tone.

We went on to talk at length about the problem I was experiencing and how much time I would be taking off. She advised me to check with our Human Resources department for the proper medical forms to fill out. We also agreed that if I felt okay, I could work at home while I was resting and building up my strength. I was so gratefully to have a manager who understood what I was going through, and supported my decision. After I left the meeting, I called my husband and told him about the decision I had made. I wish I had made this decision earlier.

That evening I talked with one of the other managers in our department, and we came up with a solution on how to manage my area while I was out on leave.

The following day I notified my staff that we would be having a meeting at 10:30 A.M. I had already talked to my two senior staff members about my intentions. I started the meeting off with light talk about how everyone was there except one team member who had the flu.

"It's good to see everyone here. The reason I called this meeting is to tell you that I am taking a 30 to 60 days leave to take care of a medical condition. My last day will be Friday." I said as I looked around the table at the team I cared so much above.

"You should have left a long time ago." John Said.

"I know."

I explained to my team about the arrangement and the manager they will be reporting to. I felt the tension in the room and made light talk again.

Then out of the blue Jeff said. "You're not coming back are you?"

"Jeff! Of course I'll be back. Where else will I go?" I asked him. On that note I ended the meeting.

I left work on Friday after talking with my team and hugging everyone. It was a sad day for me as I walked out the front door. It was almost as if I would not be coming back.

That weekend I concentrated on making a concrete decision about the course of treatment I was going to take. I was eating better and doing more exercise. The vitamins and iron pills were helping and this was proven through the tests when I only had light bleeding. I had not done the complete herbal treatment, but the parsley and kelp did help some with the heavy bleeding. But all of this was not enough I still bled heavily, and was anemic and tired most of the time.

I had studied extensive information about fibroid tumors from the Internet, TV, the newspaper and talking to others experiencing the same problems. In September, one of my friends had given me a newspaper clipping on Uterine Artery Embolization. I kept the paper in my briefcase. I pulled the paper out and read the article over and over again. This looked like a promising alternate to a hysterectomy and some of the other treatments. One thing I learned is I will have to make the decision about how I wanted my fibroids treated.

I think I wanted my doctors to tell me what to do besides taking iron pills. The same as they would if I had a heart condition, or a foot condition. I wanted to hear. "Jean, this is what we need to do to correct the condition." I didn't get the answer I wanted so desperately to hear. I wanted my doctor to make a decision for me. Sadly for me, this would not happen.

I reflected on everything I had learned during my research. I felt like a fibroid doctor still searching for answers. I was angry with myself and the doctors for not telling me how to prevent the growth of fibroids when they discovered I had them at age twenty six. Why didn't the doctors remove the tumors when they were smaller and not causing any problems? Why doctors wait until the tumors are causing problems like pain and heavy bleeding before any type of treatment is recommended? I didn't have the answer.

Bloody Monday Fibroid Tumors....My Ordeal

I had learned that fibroids are noncancerous growths that normally develop on the wall, and the outside of the uterus, although they can develop in other areas. The tumors are common in African-American women and up to fifty percent of African-American women, at some point have fibroid tumors. It is interesting that only ten to twenty percent of women suffer with any symptoms from fibroids. I fell in that ten to twenty percent.

I looked at all of the materials I had gathered. I limited myself to four treatments. Hysterectomy was the last option for me. My uterus was in good condition, and it did not make sense to have a perfectly good organ removed, because of fibroid tumors. Would I remove my leg, because it had a fibroid tumor? The answer will always be no. I would make a decision to cut the fibroid tumor off and keep the good leg.

My options included the following treatment:

- Totally change my lifestyle. Go to a more natural diet and continue with a good exercise program. Initially I will have to struggle through each monthly cycle, regardless of the length, lose the blood, and build it back up with iron pills. Hopefully, losing weight and not eating the things that cause the fibroids to grow will help control the bleeding. I was hoping that menopause would come soon and shrink the fibroids naturally. How much longer will it take for me to go through menopause two, three, ten years?

- Hysterocopy or laparoscope procedure where the uterus is filled with a liquid or gas to expand the uterus allowing the doctor to see with a light that is attached to the instrument. Small instruments are inserted through the hysteroscope to remove or reduce the size of the fibroids. In my case six weeks of hormone treatment would be needed to shrink the fibroids to about the size of a six weeks fetus to have this procedure done. I didn't want to take the hormone therapy to shrink the tumors.

- Uterine Artery Embolization was my next choice if the Hysterocopy or laparoscope procedure did not work or the bleeding became uncontrollable. This is a fairly new procedure in the United States. From my reading it has been available in the United States since 1996. Uterine Artery Embolization shrinks fibroid tumors by cutting off their blood supply. Using X-ray equipment, the radiologist threads a catheter through a small cut in the groan area to access the femoral arteries. Then small particles of polyvinyl alcohol is released into the blood vessels that are connected to the tumor blocking the blood supply, thus killing or shrinking the tumor!

- My next choice was to have the fibroids removed through myomectomy or laser surgery. This procedure would remove the fibroids without removing the uterus.

The next thing I had to do was find a gynecologist I felt comfortable with. I wanted a doctor who respected my choices and understood how I felt, regardless of how common fibroids are to black women. I didn't want to be sent home with a handful of pamphlets. I wanted my doctor to talk to me and explain everything about my condition to me.

I also needed to have the full support of my family and friends. I need to talk about my condition, and I need them to listen to me even if I talk about the same thing over and over again. And, I do talk and talk about my condition over and over again. Talking is so important to me as I am coping with this problem.

Bloody Monday Fibroid Tumors....My Ordeal

Looking for the right doctor wasn't easy. I felt as if I had hit a brick wall. I had seen two gynecologists and felt that I was not getting enough support from them medically or emotionally. I asked for recommendations and went to the HMO book to look for another doctor. It was so important to me to have a doctor who was willing to develop a medical relationship with me when it came to managing my health! My primary doctor was excellent when it came to caring for me. It would be nice if he could manage all of my problems.

That night I talked to my husband. "I am feeling better. The vitamins, herbs and iron pills are working and but I am still weak and anemic most of the time." I told him.

He just looked at me as I sat up in the bed. "Well, I am going to try to build up my blood count and look into having the Uterine Artery Embolization procedure done." I showed him the article in the paper.

"This is a new procedure. Do you think you want to do this?" He said as he glanced at the paper.

At that point, I felt that he really did not fully understand what I am going through. This is a problem that the majorities of women silently suffer and keep to themselves. Most women continue to go to work, take care of their families, and perform duties we are required to do in our weaken conditions as if nothing is wrong. I turned over and went to sleep.

January 18th, I visited my primary doctor to get a blood count and maybe a recommendation for a new gynecologist.

The doctor came into the room and said. "What's bothering you today?"

"Well, I came to get a blood count and to see if the iron pills are working." I told him.

"Okay. How are you doing with the fibroids?" He asked.

"Well, I have been bleeding almost continuously for the last six months and I want to know what gynecologist you would recommend." I asked him.

"You have? Fibroids are more of a nuisance for women, but at the same time it can be a very serious condition requiring extensive treatment." He said as he wrote down the name of the gynecologist on a piece of paper and gave it to me.

"Call this doctor. I heard she is really good," he said.

"Oh I will. I need someone who will work closer with me."

The doctor and I chatted about a few other things, including my weight. After he left the room, I went to the lab to have blood tests done. Getting the test results back would be key to the next step I would take.

I decided to look up the doctor mentioned in the newspaper article about Uterine Artery Embolization and give him a call to hopefully discuss the procedure.

I found two doctors with the same name in the phone book, at the same hospital. I decided to call the first one, and to my surprise it was the right one. I asked the receptionist if it was possible for me to talk to him. She said yes. I then asked the nurse about a referral for a gynecologist. She was very pleasant and gave me the name of one of the gynecologist practicing at the clinic. She took my information and said the doctor would call me back.

Well, the doctor did call me back. For two days the doctor tried to reach me and I missed both calls. I tried without success to reach him during those two days. I noticed that he called around 10:30 A.M. The third day I waited until 10:30 A.M. and called him. The receptionist paged him and he came to the phone.

"Hi Dr. Baine. This is Jean. I called about the Uterine Artery Embolization procedure. I just wanted to talk to you about it." I said in a nervous voice.

"I'm here to help you. Are you having the normal problems with fibroids? Heavy bleeding, Cramps, Anemic, Tiredness?" He asked.

"Yes, I am having all of that." I told him.

"Lots of women suffer with this problem. Well, the procedure is quite simple, but there are some complications involved as with any surgery." He explained.

"I know, but I think this procedure is something that I might want to try." I told him.

We talked for another five minutes about the procedure and some of he risks that could even include death as with any other major surgery. He gave me some tests that were needed before he could perform the surgery. The test included a complete exam by my gynecologist, and an endometrail biopsy to rule out anything else that may be causing the bleeding. Because my ultrasound was done over six months ago, another one would have to be done before the procedure could be preformed.

One thing the doctor told me, I had not read in the Internet articles or in the health books was disturbing. The doctor explained to me that after the Uterine Artery Embolization procedure is completed, the dead tissues from fibroids may drop off and pass from the uterus, pretty much like having a small baby delivered without the pain. He went on to explain that sometimes this dead tissue may get stuck in the uterus and the gynecologist will have to remove it. At the end of the conversation the doctor took my address to send me an information package on the procedure. He explained that he sent this package to all of his patients before the procedure is performed. I thanked him for the information. I was beginning to feel more comfortable about the procedure after talking to the doctor. I was looking forward to getting the information package.

A few days later I received the information on Uterine Artery Embolization promised by Dr. Baine. I read the information and it was similar to the information I retrieved from the Internet. I was pleased with what I read and wanted to try this procedure.

Bloody Monday Fibroid Tumors....My Ordeal

On January 25th, I received the results of the blood tests in the mail. I also stopped spotting that same day. I read the test results. My primary doctor had the area with my blood count circled and wrote a note indicating that they were a little abnormal. He also wrote a note on the test results and advised me to increase my iron pills to two a day and ended the note with "Best regards." My hematocrit count was at 33 a little low. The normal range is between 35 and 46. My hemoglobin was 11. The normal range is between 12 and 15. My red blood count was 3.64. The normal range is between 3.9 and 5.20. I was waiting for the test results before I made an appointment with another gynecologist.

I did not call the gynecologist my primary doctor recommended. Instead on Friday evening, I called the gynecologist recommended by the receptionist in Dr. Baine's office. I got the receptionist's answering service and left a message for her to call me on Monday about an appointment for the following week.

I could only wonder what this doctor would be like. I was looking forward to seeing him. I was hoping that if I did get an appointment with the doctor, he would be personal, someone who talked about my problem, and was very supportive. I was even willing to take a recommendation, if he felt that Uterine Artery Embolization procedure would not be the best treatment for my condition.

An appointment with Dr. Carnes was made for February 1st, at 9:15 A.M. I was excited. The assistant taking my information was very friendly and professional. She advised me that I would have to get to the office thirty minutes before the appointment to fill out the necessary paperwork. I learned that this doctor practiced with one of the major and respected clinics in Atlanta. I was hoping and hoping that this would work out for me. This would be my third gynecologist and I did not want to look for another doctor.

Finally, February 1st, came and I went to see the new doctor. As I pulled into the parking lot I was a little nervous. I walked into the waiting room and was surprised that it was not a normal doctor's office. It was a clinic. I must have looked startled as the one of the assistant walked up to me.

"Hi. May I help you?" She asked.

"Yes, I'm here to see Dr. Carnes."

"Okay. Just sign in at the desk where the gynecology sign is. Have a seat and you'll be called in a few minutes." She said.

"Thank you," I told her.

I signed in and found a seat in the waiting room. This time I did not bring anything to read while waiting to see the doctor. I looked around the room at the other patients. The waiting room was very noisy. Just as I was making an attempt to talk to one of the other patients the assistant called me to her desk. I went through the normal routine of filling out the necessary paperwork, copying my insurance card and paying my co-pay.

After a few minutes the nurse called my name "Ms. Alexander come with me please," she said.

The nurse showed me to another less crowded waiting room and there were about six more pages of paperwork to fill out. While I while filling out the paperwork, one of the doctors came to the waiting room.

"Are you Ms. Alexander? He asked.

"Yes I am," I told him.

"I am Dr. Elps. After you finish the paperwork, I will be talking to you about your condition before you see Dr. Carnes," he told me.

"Oh good. I'll be finished soon." I said impressed. This is a first. The doctor talking to you before you complete the paperwork!

"The nurse will be back in a few minutes and she'll direct you to my office," he said.

"Okay."

I finished the paperwork and in a few minutes the nurse came back into the waiting room. I gave her the completed paperwork.

"Okay, come with me to the doctor's office. After you finish talking to the doctor we will get your weight and blood pressure."

"Do you need a urine sample?" I asked her.

"Are you having any problems, like burning or pain when you go to the bathroom?" She asked.

"No, I'm not. I just need to use the bathroom." I told her.

"We won't need to get a urine sample, if you are not having any problems. Go on to the bathroom and then come back here." She laughed.

After I came from the bathroom I stopped by the nurse's desk. She and Dr. Epps and another doctor were waiting for me.

"Ms. Alexander, come on in my office. This is Alice one of our intern doctors from the school of medicine across the street." He said as he introduced us.

"Nice to meet you." I said.

"Well, maybe we can help you," she responded.

I sat in a chair near Dr. Epps' desk and the intern sat beside me. We went over all of the paperwork I had filled out. I was feeling really comfortable with this team, and felt that maybe at last I had made a good choice in doctors.

"My understanding is that you have heavy bleeding from fibroid tumors and Dr. Baine's office recommended you to us." He said.

"Yes."

"We get a lot of referrals from other areas. I bet your gynecologist wanted to give you a hysterectomy right?" He asked.

"Yes, she did." I said.

"Well, unless needed this is the last thing we do. But I would like to explain your condition to you and go over some things with you before Dr. Carnes examine you. After the examination a recommendation will be made and you can decide what you want to do." Dr. Epps said.

Dr. Epps explained how fibroids grow and possibly where mines might be located. We went over the history of my menstrual cycle and he explained the difference procedures that were available for the treatment of fibroids. One of the things he explained was unless a hysterectomy was done all of the other procedures did not prevent the fibroids from growing back.

"I know that you are thinking about the Uterine Artery Embolzation and this is a good procedure, but it is fairly new. Because the procedure is so new we are not sure about the long term outcome. We are not sure if the fibroids will grow back down the road," he explained.

"I guess this is one of the drawbacks of having any of the procedures done because the fibroids may grow back." I said.

"That's right. One of the things you probably have not heard or read about the Uterine Artery Embolization is after the procedures the dead tissues will fall off and you are going to have a very bad and strong odor for about two months. You are going to smell like something died inside you." He looked at me seriously.

"Really?" I asked.

"Yes, you will smell bad, and there isn't anything we can do about it. But we will be able to handle any other problems you may experience after the procedure is completed." He said.

"Did your other doctor mention the Uterine Artery Embolization procedure as an option for you?" He asked.

"No. I did read that the reason this new alternative is not recommended is because the radiologist does the procedure and the gynecologist doesn't make money from it." I said.

"Yeah, that's true. You would think those guys would share the money with us. All we do is handle the problems after the procedures are done. I do want warn you that some women having this procedure do end up having an emergency hysterectomy because of complications." He said.

"I read about that in the information Dr. Baine sent me. If this is the procedure recommended. I am willing to take that risk. I will do anything to stop the heavy bleeding." I told him.

"Okay. Let's get you to an exam room and after Dr. Carnes examines you we will get another ultrasound, do the endometrial procedure and let you know something. Okay?" He said as he touched my shoulder.

Dr. Epps called the nurse and she took me to an exam room. She asked me to get totally undressed, and gave me a cloth gown to put on and it was big enough. Oh, that gown felt good! It was cool in the exam room and I would be freezing if I had on one of those paper gowns. Just as I finished undressing the nurse came back in the room and took my blood pressure and temperature. We chatted while she did her work. After she was finished she told me that the doctor would be in shortly. After about five minutes the doctor came into the exam room.

"Ms. Alexander, I hate to do this do you, but we can do your ultrasound now and you won't have to wait. We'll do the exam after you come back. Come on with me." He said.

"I don't have on any clothes." I said.

"Oh we are all family here. Here let me tie up your gown in the back." He said and tied up my gown.

"I'll need my shoes." I said, as I got off the table and put on my shoes. I held onto the gown in the back and followed Dr. Carnes down the hall.

"How far is the ultrasound lab Dr. Carnes?" I asked.

"It's right here." He said as we entered the ultrasound lab.

The technician was preparing my paperwork as we entered the room.

"How are you Ms. Alexander?" She asked.

"I guess I am okay." I told her.

"Okay have a seat in that chair and we can get started." She said.

"I've never had an ultrasound in a chair before." I said

"This is one of the ways we do them. Okay put your feet in the stirrups. I am going to let the chair back. You may feel like you are going to fall, but you won't." She laughed.

The back of the chair began to move toward the floor, as the seat of the chair moved in an upward position. The technician and I were chatting about her going to medical school to be a doctor and her children. I looked up and wondered when she would put the jelly on my stomach when I saw the long vaginal ultrasound probe.

"You're not going to use that probe are you?" I asked.

"Yes I am. It's not going to hurt." She said as she put a lubricant and a cover on the probe.

Oh well, I may as well get use to this. Maybe I'll continue to talk to her and it will be over fast. I started the conversation again about my children and she picked it up and continued to talk more about her children. After about fifteen minutes she was finished. The technician showed me a curtain to go behind and gave me some towels to cleanse the jelly from my body. Just as I finished she made a low groan.

"Oh, Ms. Alexander, Ms. Alexander. I forgot to get one picture. I thought I had it." She said.

"Oh no not again!" I said.

"Sit back on the chair. It won't take long. I promise." She said.

I sat back on the chair and watched as she prepared the probe again. She was finished in no time. Again I went back behind the curtain and cleanse the jelly from my body.

"Okay we got it that time." The technician said.

"It wasn't that bad." I said.

"No it wasn't. Okay. I'll walk you back to the exam room and get these test results to Dr. Carnes." She said.

We walked back to the exam room and I thanked her for everything. I pulled off my shoes and got on the exam table. I had already been at the doctor's office for more than an hour. I was hoping that the exam would not take long. I had been probed so much that the pelvic exams were not as embarrassing as they were before. I waited for another ten minutes before the doctor, the nurse, and the intern came into the room.

"Okay, Jean. May I call you Jean?" He asked.

"Sure." I told him.

"Let's start the exam. Put your feet here and push down to the end of the table." He instructed.

As he began to examine me he said. "Everything looks okay. Right now there's no bleeding. I am going to do a Pap smear right now, so just relax.

"Okay." I said.

"Jean, now I am going to do the endometrial procedure. It may feel a little uncomfortable. So just relax," he said.

The nurse passed the doctor the necessary instrument to do the procedure. I looked at the nurse and the intern. Suddenly the room seemed so small. I felt some pain as the doctor took small pieces of tissue from my uterus and put it in the specimen container the nurse was holding.

"I didn't get enough to do the test." The doctor said as he looked at the nurse. "Jean I am going to have to do this one more time," he said.

"Ah, I got some that time," the doctor said. "Well, Jean, not being able to get much tissue is a good indication that your uterus is okay."

"That's good to know," I said.

"Okay Jean, get dressed and come down to my office and let's discuss some things we can do to help you with this problem."

"Okay," I said.

The doctor and his assistants left the room and I got dressed in a hurry. I couldn't help but wonder what Dr. Carnes would say. I was eager to learn about the ultrasound tests and the doctor's recommendation. After I got dressed I went to the doctor's office.

"Have a seat Jean," he said.

"First let's go over the ultrasound tests. You have two fibroids inside the uterus. From experience, we have found that the position of your tumors can cause very heavy and prolonged periods. They are about fourteen weeks, the size of a three to four month fetus." He said.

"They use to be fourteen to sixteen weeks. Do you think they are shrinking?" I said.

"Well, maybe," he said.

"Let me draw you a picture showing you where your fibroids are positioned in the uterus," he said.

This is the first time a doctor has ever taken the time to explain exactly what was happening in my body. This is the picture Dr. Carnes drew for me showing where the fibroids are located in my uterus. I have two fibroids, one on each side of the uterus. I looked intensely at the picture as the doctor pointed to the different locations fibroids can grow in or on the outside of the uterus.

"Jean, I know that you would like to have the Uterine Artery Embolization, and it is a good procedure, but at this point I would not recommend it." He said.

"Why?" I asked as my hopes for a permanent solution for my problem faded.

"Well, the first thing I would recommend would be a Laparoscopy. This is a procedure where we will fill the uterus with a liquid solution and use a telescope on a small thin tool, so we can get a good look inside the uterus. Using this same tool with other instruments we shave the fibroids down. We have had a seventy-five to eighty-five percent success rate with improvement in heavy and prolonged bleeding. If this method fails then I would recommend the Uterine Artery Embolization procedure."

"What would I have to do to have the Laparoscopy procedure done?" I asked him.

"Well, we will have to shrink the fibroids down to six weeks before we can perform this procedure. I know that you took the hormone shots for two months before and it did not work. I would use a stronger hormone shot, just for six weeks to totally shut down the ovaries. You won't bleed during this time, but you will have all the symptoms of menopause," he explained.

"Hormone shots make me crazy. I really don't want to go through that again unless I absolutely have to. Is there any other way to shrink the fibroids?" I asked.

"This is the method we use and we have had great success with it. From your chart you should have a cycle in a few days. After your cycle is complete we will give you the hormone shot," he said.

"I don't know. I was trying to avoid taking the hormones. If I decide to have this procedure done will the fibroids grow back?" I asked.

"Yes they can. Jean here's my card with my assistant's name on it. I know that you have some concerns, and I want you to think it over before you make a decision. I just want to let you know that if you do decide to have the procedure it would be done here at the office. I normally perform the procedure on Fridays. This way you can be back to work on Monday," he said.

"Okay, let me think about it and I will get back with you," I said.

"Take care of yourself and continue to take the vitamins and the iron pills. Let me know what you want to do." He said as he touched me on the shoulder.

Bloody Monday Fibroid Tumors....My Ordeal

After I left the office I was both pleased and disappointed. I was pleased with the doctor and the personal care he and his staff gave me. Explaining everything to me about fibroid tumors, and procedures and medicine used to treat fibroids. I was disappointed because the Uterine Artery Embolization procedure was not the doctor's first recommendation, based on his examination. I was also disappointed that the doctor did not discuss diet or any other nutritional factors that could contribute to the grown or shrinkage of the fibroids except the estrogen produced by my body.

Driving home I thought about my doctor's visit. Regardless of what I choice to do besides taking my uterus out, the fibroids can grow back.

That day I decided not to have any of the procedures done unless absolutely necessary. I decided to change my lifestyle and stick with it. I would go to a more natural diet and exercise program. This meant that I would also have to get my weight down, struggle through the monthly cycles, regardless of the length, lose the blood, and build it back up with the iron pills.

I had earlier considered becoming a member of a weight lost program, but changed my mind because I had done this so many times before without much success. I realized that if I did not change my habits and thinking process I would not be successful regardless of what I decided to do. I was interested in more than just losing weight. I was interested in changing my lifestyle. The question is can I do this on my own? I boldly told myself yes!

On February 2nd, I pulled out my health books and started looking for a program that would be healthy and work for me. I wasn't looking for miracles, or instant results. The changes I had already made were helping my condition and I felt encouraged to do more.

I felt upbeat. I had made this decision, now the challenge was sticking with it. That very day, one of my friends called and asked me to exercise with them in the mall.

"Jean, the girls and I go walking in the mall every morning at 6:30 A.M. Do you want to join us?" She asked.

"That's too early for me!" I told her.

"Why? This is a great way to lose weight and it may even help your problem," she said.

"I know. I really do need to exercise, but that is just too early in the morning." I said.

"Okay. Let me know when you want to join us," she said.

After hanging up the phone, I sat down at the table and decided on an exercise program that was suitable for me. I decided that walking would be the best exercise for me. I wasn't good at aerobics and I wanted to start off walking about fifteen minutes a day seven days a week. I also decided to do sit ups about three times a week. I could still dance if I wanted to get in some extra exercise. I reasoned that this program should be easy enough for someone like me who is totally out of shape.

I was determined to do this life style change one day at a time. Changing my eating habits would be a bigger challenge. I had to consider the family in this change, and I had to come up with a very flexible menu. The menu had to be structured in a way that would allow my family to have the goodies they wanted, while providing me with the necessary changes I needed to make in my diet to control the growth of the fibroids.

"Ah... No more fried foods." As I thought about how much I loved fried chicken, and okra!

That day when my husband came home I approached him and said. "We are going to have a different way of eating. Well maybe not that different, but we will be eating more fresh vegetables and fruits."

"That's good. It's just what we need," he said.

I went back to my health books at my favorite spot on the dining room table, and began to put together a menu. There are a few things I knew I would have to limit on the menu. This would be Fatty fried foods, soft drinks, dairy products, beef and one thing in particular ice creams! Oh, how I love ice cream. What am I going to do without ice cream!

I started the menu off with breakfast. I am not much of a breakfast person, but I know that it is the most important meal of the day. So what will I eat for breakfast?

Breakfast would mostly consist of herbal tea, a bowl of mixed fruit, and a slice of wheat bread if desired. I had to substitute the tea for my beloved coffee.

Sample Breakfast Menus

Sliced Apples
Wheat Toast
Carrots
Herbal Tea
Water

Bran Muffin
Orange
Herbal Tea
Water

Oatmeal
Apple
Herbal Tea
Water

Mixed Fruit Bowl
Herbal Tea
Water

Sample Lunch Menus

Vegetable plate
A roll or cornbread muffin
Herbal Tea
Water

Grilled Chicken Salad
Herbal Tea
Water

Vegetable Soup
Fruit bowl
Herbal Tea
Water

Chicken Salad Sandwich
Light Mayo, Lettuce,
Tomatoes
Apple
Herbal Tea
Water

Sample Dinner Menus

Grilled Salmon
Steamed Broccoli
Rice
Carrots
Herbal Tea
Water

Herbal Roasted Chicken
Baked Sweet Potatoes
Spinach
Herbal Tea
Water

Broccoli
Corn
Tossed Salad
Herbal Tea
Water

Turkey Lasagna
Tossed Salad
Herbal Tea
Water

Sample Snacks

Orange
Apples
Bananas
Pop-Corn

Jell-O
Cantaloupe
Other Fruits

All of the meats on menu are to be baked or grilled. The vegetable would be steamed or stirred fried using my favorite Canola oil. Herbal tea would be my choice for drinks. I decided to have my choice of salad dressings as a treat as long as I limited the portions. I made a rule. If I ate meat for lunch I will not eat meat for dinner. Cutting back on the salt and using lots of herbal seasoning would be used when preparing foods. I also made a decision that I would eat only when I am hungry and not because it was time to eat. The hardest part for me will be drinking at least sixty-four ounces of water a day. I am not very fond of water, and it is going to be a task to drink sixty-four ounces of it. But, I would take it one step at a time increasing the water intake a little at a time.

Bloody Monday Fibroid Tumors....My Ordeal

I started my new way of eating the very same day. My family wasn't too thrilled with the way I seasoned the food. I had to add a little more to their food but I kept mines the same.

One evening I was out with one of my friends and she began to talk about an herbal presentation she was having at her house. I was interested and was hoping she would invite me, without me inviting myself.

Finally she asked. "Jean we're having an herbal presentation at my house tonight. I thought you might be interested in coming. It's Saturday at 5:30 P.M. Do you think you can come?"

"Yes, I'll love to. I've been looking at a cleansing program, but I don't want the one where they use the liquid solution to cleanse your colon. I am looking for something that is gentle on my system, and takes about a week or more to work," I told her.

"Come to the presentation Saturday and tell the girl what you are looking for. I am sure they have something like that," she said.

"I'll be there." I said as I got out of the car and headed for the house.

I could not wait until Saturday. My friend gave me some information about the company. As I read I learned that their products were made from natural foods. I was really interested.

On Saturday, I went to the presentation. There were about 10 other people present. I listened intensely at the presentation and tasted most of the herbal teas that the speaker served to us. The herbal tea tasted really good! The speaker informed us to always check with our doctors before starting any new cleansing or diet program. We sat through an hour long presentation and finally it was coming to an end.

"Are there any questions?" She asked.

"Which product would you recommend using first?" I asked.

"Well, I would start with the cleansing package first. It's an all food product with this wonderful tea. It is not harsh and you can use it alone with a regular and balanced diet." She said.

I looked at the cleansing program. It included nutritional bars, herbal supplements, herbal teas and a natural sweetener. You could substitute the nutritional bars for one or two of your meals, and take the herbs and drink the cleansing herbal teas at least three times a day. This sounded okay, and the products contained the same ingredient I could get at the health food store.

I decided to give it a try for one week and one week only. I filled out my order and gave it to the speaker at the table.

"I would like to order the cleansing package. I am going to try it for a week and see what happens," I told her.

"This is a good choice. You will love it. Call me and let me know after you finish this. If you want more or want to go to the basic program you can order it yourself. All of the information you need will be included when you receive your order. You should receive your order in about two days," she told me.

I stayed at my friend's house for another hour and talked with the other guests and some who had tried the program. Finally I headed home. The next week I waited patiently for the cleansing package to come. In the meantime I needed to get in touch with my primary doctor to let him know that I was going to try the natural way to control the fibroids growth, get the weight down, and the tell him about the additional herbs and teas I was taking. I called my primary doctor's office but he was on vacation. I'll tell him about these changes when I see him again for my next checkup.

The cleansing package came on Thursday and I decided to start it on Saturday. I waited patiently for Saturday to some. To my surprise and horror, Friday night February 16th my cycle began. I had spent a glorious twenty-three days without bleeding. At first I started to put off starting the cleansing program, but decided that I would stick to my schedule.

I still feared going out when my cycle was on and this would be the perfect time to start the cleansing program. The program was scheduled to last for five days. I was a little nervous, because I had two things to deal with, the introduction of a new cleansing program and my monthly cycle. I didn't know what to expect.

"I am out for the weekend." I told my husband. "I am starting this new cleansing program tomorrow. Maybe you should try it."

"No, that's okay. I don't need cleaning out. I am just fine the way I am," he said.

"Okay. If it works, I am going to order the other teas and add them to my diet," I told him.

"Help yourself! I just don't need any additional help in that area." He convincingly said.

I had been free from fear for twenty three days and now it was returning. I dreaded what would happen in the next few days. Fear gripped my heart. Although I was not bleeding heavy, out of habit, I found myself sitting in the chair near the bathroom in my bedroom.

Bloody Monday Fibroid Tumors....My Ordeal

Day one on the cleansing program didn't do much, but days two through five really did what the product had promised. I had a good cleansing.

Days one through five of my cycle were very light with no clotting at all. I didn't have to stay at home but I was still afraid to venture out to far from home.

I felt that day six would be different as I got out of bed. I noticed that the bleeding was heavy with moderate clotting. I was scared. I had hoped that all the changes I had made would help. I prayed that the bleeding would not be too bad. To my surprise after about two hours the bleeding and clotting slowed to normal. I could not help but wonder how long my cycle last?

I made up my mind not to stress myself out about how long this would go on. I was pleased so far that the bleeding was not too bad. For the first time I was having somewhat of a normal cycle and if it stayed on longer than normal, I would have to accept that. I was more concerned with controlling the amount of bleeding. A calmness came over me and I felt more in control of the situation. The fear began to slowly leave me.

I was very pleased with the cleansing products. I decided to order more herbal teas and supplements. The teas are wonderful, and I liked the fact that I could drink them daily. The herbal supplements are different because they will assist in keeping my body balanced by providing me with the fiber and other nutrients I may miss in my daily diet.

After reading the information, I decided that the cleansing teas and the herbal supplements was the only two items I needed. There are other products I can get, but I had to choose what I think is best for me now. I like this product. This is the first time in six months that my period was almost normal.

I had an unusually long break from February to March and did not have another period until April. I had not missed any days from work for menstrual related problems since my return to work on February 26th. On April 2nd, my period came and I felt that old familiar fear creep up in me again. I was scared. I still had not gained total truth in my body. My daughter was on spring break, so I decided to stay at home with her. To my surprise, I had a normal cycle. There was no excessive bleeding or pain. I was so thankful.

After such a good month in April, I was encouraged even more to continue to drink the herbal teas and stayed as close as I could to my new eating plan and exercise program. I had not lost too much weight, but all of my clothes are fitting better. I could fit in clothes that were too small for me just a few months ago.

May and June proved to be excellent months. My cycle was normal! There were no clots, no need for heavy pads or those super plus tampons.

Since I started the cleansing program, drinking the herbal teas and taking the supplements I have not taken any other vitamins, herbs or iron pills since February.

I went back to my primary doctor for a check up and blood tests. I couldn't wait for the results. It would take a week for the results to return.

A week later I went back to the doctor for the blood test results. After checking in at the front desk, I was shown to the exam room. I sit on the exam table and nervously waited for the doctor.

The doctor walked in the room smiling. "Well Jean, good news. All of your blood tests are normal. Your blood count is really good. It is near normal."

I let out a sigh of relief. "Oh, that's good news."

"Are you still taking the iron pills?" He asked.

"No. I am not. I changed my diet and I have not been feeling tired." I told him.

"Okay." He said.

"What about the heavy bleeding?" He asked.

"Well for the last three months the bleeding has been manageable. In April and May I had pretty normal periods." I told him.

"That's good. I'm glad to see that you've changed your diet, and it's working for you. By the way your blood pressure is normal too." He informed me.

The doctor examined me and told me that everything appeared to be okay. He wanted to see me in three months. He didn't have any questions or too much to say about the changes I had made in my life.

Although I have made changes, I still struggle with controlling the sweets in my diet. I love chocolates, ice cream, and hard candy. I have cut down considerable, but I still eat them from time to time.

Overall I am still making progress. I am convinced that the changes I have made in my lifestyle have played a big role in controlling the heavy bleeding and hopefully the growth of the fibroids.

Bloody Monday Fibroid Tumors....My Ordeal

I have confidence that my next checkup with the gynecologist will be favorable. I don't feel the pressure against my bladder or in the lower part of my body that I felt just a few months ago. I made an appointment to see Dr. Carnes.

On June 26th, I went to the doctor. I checked in at the desk and waited for my name to be called. After about ten minutes the nurse called my name.

"Ms. Alexander. Come on back with me." She said. As we walked toward the doctor's office Dr. Carnes met us.

"Come on in Jean. Are you still having the heavy bleeding?" He asked.

"No, not since February. I decided to change my diet and exercise more and it appears to be working." I told him.

"So, you're doing better?" He asked.

"Yes, I am. This is what I am doing. First I cut out the coffee. This was a struggle but I did it. I started drinking herbal teas. I did a five day cleansing program. Then I started to eat more vegetables and fruits." I said.

"Well, changing the eating habits may have helped, but exercise does not have much effect on fibroids. Okay let's examine you." He said.

The doctor walked with me to the exam room and instructed me to get undressed from the waist down and left the room.

A few minutes later the doctor and nurse came back in the exam room. The nurse took my blood pressure and said it was okay. The doctor began to examine me.

"Okay we are finished. I have some good news. The fibroids have not grown any. They are about the same size." He said.

"That is good news." I said.

"Jean, we doctors normally don't say what I am about to say." He said.

"What is it?" I asked him.

"What you are doing appears to be working for you. We recommend all of these procedures, but you have found a way to control the bleeding through diet and exercise. If it is working for you keep doing it." He said.

"I will." I said.

"I want you to know that it doesn't matter how large or small the fibroids are they can cause heavy bleeding, or they may not have any symptoms at all. I'm happy for you." He said.

"It's been really hard for me, Dr. Carnes. I still have the fear of heavy periods. I still don't fully trust my body, but I am going to stick to the changes I've made." I told him.

"Jean if you should ever need me for anything, just give me a call." He said and touched me on the shoulder.

"I will." I said as I watched him walk out of the exam room.

I got dressed and danced around in the exam room. Although the changes I made are working, I have not ruled out surgery if needed in the future. I find it amazing that the few changes I made in my lifestyle resulted in big changes in the way my body is reacting to uterine fibroid tumors.